Cosmetic Surgery Without Fear

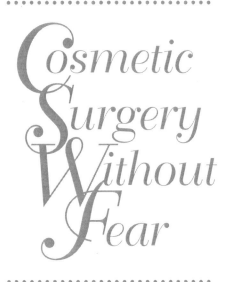

Cosmetic Surgery Without Fear

*How to Make
Safe Choices
and
Informed Decisions*

Patricia Burgess

COSMETIC SURGERY CONSULTANTS
ATLANTA, GEORGIA

Cosmetic Surgery Consultants
4343 Shallowford Road, Suite B–5
Marietta, GA 30062
Phone: (770) 552-3223   Fax: (770) 552-9054
E-mail: explore@cscfirst.com
www.safecosmeticsurgery.com

Individual Sales. This book is available through most bookstores or can be ordered directly from Cosmetic Surgery Consultants at the address above.

Quantity Sales. Special discounts are available on quantity purchases by corporations, associations, and other organizations. For details, contact the "Special Sales Department" at the Cosmetic Surgery Consultants address above.

Printed in the United States of America

Publisher's Cataloging-in-Publication
(Provided by Quality Books, Inc.)

Burgess, Patricia Anne.
    Cosmetic surgery without fear : how to make
safe choices and informed decisions / Patricia
Burgess. -- 1st ed.
    p. cm.
    Includes bibliographical references and index.
    ISBN: 0-9667630-0-9

    1. Surgery, Plastic--Popular works.
    I. Title.

RD118.B87 1999   617.9'5
                                   QBI99-770

Editorial Services: PeopleSpeak
Interior design/typesetting: Graffolio Design and Typesetting
Cover design: George Foster, Foster & Foster

Every attempt has been made to present accurate and timely information. We have used many sources, including our own professional and personal experiences, to compile the information found in this guide. The field of plastic, cosmetic, and reconstructive surgery is constantly changing, which will account for many of the changes in references, resources, information, statistics, technology, approaches, or techniques that no doubt will occur by the time this book is purchased or read. Many individuals, scientists, and medical, legal, and healthcare professionals may voice their own findings and opinions, which may differ significantly from those included in this guide. Therefore, nothing contained herein should constitute an absolute with regard to this subject matter or be considered a substitute for legal, medical, or psychological advice.

Distributed by Access Publishers Network
6893 Sullivan Road, Grawn, MI 49637
(800) 345-0096

To

Rona Hertz Mazer

1954 – 1999

Who always saw the possibilities

Contents

Preface

One little tip, one fear allayed, or one understandable explanation makes a world of difference to a patient's cosmetic surgery experience. Thinking about cosmetic surgery is exciting yet can be overwhelming. There are many considerations—risks, physician selection, preparation for surgery, recovery, and more.

To make your cosmetic surgery decision a bit less daunting, *Cosmetic Surgery without Fear* was compiled as a comprehensive resource guide. We wanted to provide timely, useful tips and information that you can employ immediately—even before you go to your first physician consultation. The objective is to inform and educate you so that you can avoid the problems we all fear. Patient consultants—who have personally undergone cosmetic surgery as well as extensive training, including observing surgeries performed by some of the best surgeons in the country—contributed to the information contained in this book. Additionally, all of the information about the procedures and other informational sections has been reviewed for clinical accuracy by cosmetic surgeons (both plastic and reconstructive and facial plastic surgeons).

No one can ever guarantee the exact results of surgery. However, your chances of success are greatly increased when you understand the process and become proactive in your search for the aesthetic enhancements of which you have always dreamed.

We have designed this book so that you can utilize it through every stage of your cosmetic surgery experience, from deciding which physician to choose through your recovery. We recommend that you read the information section first so that you will be aware of all the factors that go into making an informed decision. Then proceed to the specific procedure in which you are interested. At each phase of your cosmetic surgery journey, refer back to the section that addresses the topic you are researching.

We are aware that some of the information may seem redundant, especially if you are researching several procedures. However, as you progress through the process, we know that your focus will change at each stage along the way. For example, when you are preparing for your initial consultations with physicians, you will be concentrating on the section "Questions to Ask the Doctor" and not be concerned with detailed recovery information or patient tips. Additionally, we feel that many points need to be repeated.

Cosmetic surgery is an exciting and rewarding decision when entered into wisely. We wish you much success. Please let us know about your journey, experiences, and results as you explore the possibilities.

Note: Throughout the book we have chosen to use the terms "he," "him," and "his" when referring to physicians and "she," "her," and "hers" when referring to patients. Our intent is to be clear and less cumbersome with the verbiage in this book, not to be exclusionary. Additionally, we have chosen to use the word "procedure," even though we realize you may choose to have multiple procedures performed at one time.

Acknowledgments

A heartfelt THANK YOU to the following wonderful individuals:

- Susan Monteleone-Laird, for her dedication to this project, her diligent research and writing, and her capacity to translate everyone's thoughts into the written word.

- Sandra N. Page, R.N., for her expertise, both clinically and from the patient's perspective (she has donated her body to science while still alive).

- The plastic and reconstructive surgeons, as well as the facial plastic and reconstructive surgeons on our medical advisory board who contributed their time and knowledge to ensure we provided clinically accurate information.

- And a special thank you to two other members of our advisory board who gave us so much of their time, shared their resources, and were always available to answer any questions:

  Alison O'Neil, MH/HS Esthetician and Medical Rehabilitation Specialist

  Pat Tucker, Patient Advocate

- Samantha Rosenberg, of DVR Designs, for her pursuit of excellence while preparing this manuscript for final layout and design.

- Nancy Clemmer, for her assistance with editing and proofreading.

- Sharon Goldinger, of People Speak—Copyeditor and more. Sharon's passion for the publishing business, fervent interest in the success of her clients, and work ethic, as evidenced by inhuman hours on the west coast to accommodate us in the east, has been a joy and pleasure to know.

- Sue Knopf, of Graffolio, for our book design, layout, and typesetting. We thank her for her patience, reliability, responsiveness, extraordinary thoroughness, talent, and willingness to work with us even when we create confusion.

- John Lindberg, of Access Publishers Network, for seeing potential in this project in its earliest, roughest stage and for spending much time sharing his knowledge and helping to develop the possibilities.

- Tami De Palma, Kim Dushinski, and Bradley James of MarketAbility who also see the possibilities, seem to have unlimited energy, love what they do, and do it well.

- Apolonia Fortino, Center for Inner Work, who waters the seeds of magnificence in all who cross her path.
- Gary Zielinski, my husband, who is always there and never doubts.

What You Don't Know Can Hurt You

We have all heard the horror stories about cosmetic surgery, but somehow we believe nothing can happen to us. When we take the time to become informed, we greatly increase the chance of a successful outcome. Information is knowledge and knowledge is power. Becoming empowered helps you make informed choices.

By observing the medical industry, we noticed a few interesting facts about referral companies, information sources, and people's ideas about the seriousness of cosmetic surgery. Cosmetic surgery referral companies—in the form of telephone or Internet referral sources—appear to be more interested in the prospective patient's zip code than in the procedures being contemplated. The criterion these companies use to determine the quality of the surgeons is "board certification"—a good start, but not nearly enough.

Most of the stories we hear regarding problems with plastic surgery involve surgeons who are board certified. A board-certified surgeon who is impaired because of substance abuse or who is "trained" to perform nose reshaping but only performs two a year would not be a suitable candidate for a physician for most of us. However, no referral sources currently available screen for quality and accountability in cosmetic surgery. Most of the consultants at referral companies are former patients themselves, who tout as their credentials the fact that they have "been there." But prospective patients should be looking for a lot more than empathy from someone who wants to advise them about the wonders of cosmetic surgery.

Much of the information in books, advertisements, and on the Internet comes directly from physicians or organizations supporting physicians. Consequently, it often has a "marketing angle" or a degree of bias. The process of gathering and sorting through this information can be so overwhelming that a prospective patient may not undertake the task, not from the lack of interest but from a lack of time or energy.

Finally, a common notion about this field of healthcare is that cosmetic surgery is not "real" surgery. This is a serious misconception. People talk a lot about "lunchtime lifts" and other quick fixes in ways that tend to minimize the reality of cosmetic surgery.

For the next several pages we will provide some reality: a compilation of notions or ideas about cosmetic surgery that you may or may not have considered. The idea here is not to scare you but to challenge you and get you thinking. If you learn just one morsel of information that you weren't aware of before, then your time and investment in this book will have been well spent.

Did You Know?

 It is a startling fact, but true—anyone with a medical degree can perform cosmetic surgery, whether or not he's had specific training. For many, hearing about a doctor operating without experience acts as a wake-up call. We might ask, "How can this be?" We live in such a regulated society—why wouldn't this segment of healthcare be as regulated as the rest?

Cosmetic surgery is less regulated than other kinds of healthcare for two reasons. First, cosmetic surgery for aesthetic purposes is generally elective. When there is no insurance component and the surgery is not being paid for in a "pooled" manner (such as by a health or car insurance policy), it isn't a "public" issue. It is a private transaction between patient and doctor. The regulators aren't interested.

Second, as a result of managed care, many physicians feel that their fees have been excessively lowered and they are trying to find ways to recoup their losses. The only remaining medical specialty in which doctors obtain full pay, without managed care interference, is cosmetic surgery. For this reason, an increasing number of physicians' advertisements now assert expertise in procedures in which the doctors may not have had specific training.

When evaluating your physician's credentials, be sure to ask about board certification in the physician's specialty and make inquiries concerning specific training, expertise, and licensure (See "Physician Screening and Selection" on page 26). As an individual you can make some verifications, and it is imperative that you follow through with what is available to you. (See "Data Available to Individuals" on page 29.)

Did You Know?

A doctor may have sanctions against him in one state and still practice in another. The public has no way of knowing. Currently, the public cannot access the kinds of databases that house information on malpractice history and disciplinary actions. Some information is posted on the Internet, but its reliability and accuracy are in question at this time.

In most cases, the signature of the physician in question will be necessary to authorize the release of this type of information. And even if you can get this release, you will still need additional identifying information, such as the physician's social security number and birth date, to make sure you are evaluating the correct "John Smith, M.D."

Healthcare organizations have access to a lot of the information that the public does not. For example, the National Practitioner Data Bank (NPDB), which reports sanctions, license suspensions, limitations, and other disciplinary actions, is open to health maintenance organizations (HMOs), preferred provider organizations (PPOs), and other healthcare entities but is closed to the general public. In 1986 Congress passed the Health Care Quality Improvement Act, which established the NPDB database but banned the public from access to its contents. Certain consumer groups are lobbying for it to be opened to the public. The American Medical Association (AMA), on the other hand, has made a resolution to destroy the data bank.

Take the time to gather as much information as you can from the physician, including his schooling and board certification status. You can call the medical licensing board in your state to see if your doctor's license is active and in good standing. All states differ as to the kinds of information they will release over the telephone to an individual. Some will post disciplinary actions; some will not.

These are tough questions to ask a physician, but if you are bold enough, consider asking the doctor to provide his social security number and birth date. Let him know that you plan to take advantage of the information available to you and that you wouldn't want to mistake another doctor's information for his. These identifiers may then make the information on the Internet a little more reliable. (See "Physician Screening and Selection, Data Available to Individuals" on page 29.)

Did You Know?

Another doctor or an associate could perform your surgery without your consent, unless you state in writing the name of the doctor you have chosen. You may have heard the recent concerns about "substitute surgeons," as featured on programs like *20/20* and *Dateline*. It's true. If you do not specify the physician's name you have chosen on your consent forms, you risk the possibility that someone you did not authorize will perform the surgery.

Many doctors have associates who are in training and who may assist the primary physician with the surgery. This is fine, but make sure that the primary surgeon is always present and fully involved and not relinquishing his duties to his student.

Substitute surgeons are a problem that is easily overlooked, but one that is also easily remedied. Request that the name(s) of the doctor(s) performing surgery be placed on your consent forms. Ask if there will be an associate assisting with the surgery. If so, include language that states there will be full and primary involvement by your chosen doctor. Absolutely nothing is wrong with asking this of your doctor. Of course, you will have evaluated your principal surgeon's credentials prior to this.

Did You Know?

If a facility is not accredited, it is not required to have monitoring or lifesaving equipment on the premises. According to the Federated Ambulatory Surgery Association, a survey completed in 1997 of 2,328 surgical centers (including centers other than for plastic surgery) indicated that only 52 percent were accredited by one of the accreditation entities. That means that 48 percent did not opt to go through the more rigorous accreditation process. It is most likely that the 48 percent did have some sort of site inspection by the respective state, but not necessarily. According to these statistics, your chances of being treated at a non-accredited facility are approximately 50 percent.

Today, most cosmetic surgeries take place in an outpatient facility—one that is part of a hospital complex or owned and operated by the surgeon. Accreditation organizations exist whose sole function is to make certain that these facilities meet high quality and safety standards. (See "Surgical Facility Accreditation" on page 32.)

We spend so much time and consideration on *who* is going to perform the surgery, but we neglect to ask *where* it will take place. If a surgical facility is accredited, it is required to have either an anesthesiologist who is a medical doctor or a nurse anesthetist, along with monitoring and resuscitation equipment. Tragedies have occurred where there was no monitoring or resuscitation equipment on site, which resulted in the untimely and preventable deaths of cosmetic surgery patients. These are the stories that all of us fear. Just a simple question about the status of facility accreditation for the location you are considering may be all that is needed to avoid a needless medical catastrophe.

Unfortunately, submitting to accreditation by these groups is completely voluntary. If a doctor owns his own surgical suite, he could choose not to spend the money and time necessary to undergo this process. It is a rigorous process— so if accreditation does exist, or the facility is willing to seek accreditation, it is a sign that the doctor/facility you have chosen is safety and quality minded.

Ask to see the facility's certification. If there is only state certification, with no certificate from the specialty accreditation organizations (see "Surgical Facility Accreditation" on page 32), you may wish to schedule your surgery elsewhere.

Did You Know?

There could be surgical options or approaches that are better suited to your case that have not been disclosed by your doctor. This is partly because physicians' approaches, training, and comfort level with specific procedures are often very different. Physicians tend to feel strongly proprietary about the procedures that they perform on a regular basis. When we visit any physician, we must remember that he is marketing his particular training and expertise. Generally, there is nothing right or wrong about this, but you need to be aware of what your choices are and in what circumstances they make sense. Sometimes you'll even get conflicting information. You would be well served to become informed about the surgical options for a given procedure and then ask your doctors during your interviews why they would or would not recommend that option.

Getting conflicting information is a good indicator that you should visit two to three doctors. This way you may gain consensus among at least two physicians.

If all of the opinions conflict, continue visiting carefully selected doctors until there is some measure of agreement. This is just prudent, good judgment.

An example is the three surgical options generally used for a brow lift: (1) coronal or temporal, (2) endoscopic, or (3) in the natural creases of the forehead (usually performed on men). For a woman, the choice is usually either a coronal brow lift or an endoscopic lift. The coronal or temporal lift uses a large incision behind the hairline, most often from ear to ear. The endoscopic technique involves three to five tiny incisions just behind the hairline. If someone has a tendency toward thinning hair, the coronal scar could become visible, with age. If you were not aware of the options, and your doctor was proficient in only one of these approaches, the likelihood is that you would not be given a choice. (See "Procedure" on page 125 for surgical options in each procedure.)

Typically, each procedure has more than one approach, especially as the field of aesthetic surgery continues to grow and new advances are introduced. You must be aware of all possibilities.

Becoming informed of your choices is critical if you are to have an intelligent and healthy exchange with your doctors. Visiting several doctors, reading books, using a consulting firm, and searching the Internet can provide you with information about available options. The decisions you make will then be the best ones for you.

Did You Know?

Political and philosophical differences among various specialties can create a great deal of confusion for the prospective patient, especially if those differences result in one doctor disparaging another. When this happens, it could sound as if a doctor is speaking poorly about another doctor's quality of care. Often these remarks reflect a personality clash and not necessarily the quality of services. Most prospective patients see critical comments for what they are (inappropriate and unprofessional) and feel that such comments reflect negatively on their source. The doctor you choose should be educating you as to what he does, not discussing what others are doing, except to share additional options. Here we get to see that physicians are human, too!

The field of plastic and cosmetic surgery has become highly competitive. Some doctors (and organizations) believe they are the only ones who should perform certain procedures. This rather narrow view could be construed as self-serving and would deprive the public of quality services by doctors who truly do have expertise in certain areas. On the other hand, some surgeons do operate outside of their scope of practice. For example, a gynecologist performing breast augmentations or a dermatologist offering to perform a rhinoplasty (nose reshaping) would be physicians to avoid.

You should be familiar with the different specialties within the field of cosmetic surgery. These specialties may include plastic and reconstructive surgeons, facial plastic surgeons (who are generally trained as ear, nose and throat [ENT] doctors and take additional training in facial plastic surgery), cosmetic dermatologists, ophthalmologists who specialize in occuloplastic surgery (which encompasses cosmetic and reconstructive procedures of the eye area), and others. All of these specialty groups have contributed a great deal to cosmetic surgery as we know it today. By responding to advertisements or picking a doctor out of the Yellow Pages, many patients find their way to all of these different doctors, yet most patients are unaware of the differences in board certifications, training, or scope of practice.

Without taking the time to research the differences mentioned above, a patient really does risk choosing the wrong doctor. However, don't dismiss a doctor's appropriateness for you just because another doctor criticizes him. Listen carefully, sometimes between the lines, and screen each surgeon for his particular training and experience.

Find out what specialty your chosen doctor works within when you're verifying his other credentials. After you have taken personal responsibility to become informed, trust your judgment. Much of the doctor-patient relationship is based on effective communication. You must feel that you are heard and being understood. This connection with your surgeon cannot be qualified or quantified, but it must be factored in as part of the overall physician selection process.

Did You Know?

We spend more time contemplating the purchase of an automobile than we do researching a cosmetic surgeon. We seem to care more about what we drive around in than what we walk around in. Why do we select a car more carefully than a surgeon? Perhaps because the process of buying a car is a little more familiar? The car-buying experience can be agonizing, yet we subject ourselves to it because we want to get the best possible car for our money. Sometimes we get so caught up in a car's look, options, status, and how we feel about driving the car that we make hasty decisions. A cosmetic surgery decision is often more an emotional decision than a medical one and could be likened to buying a car. However, you generally get rid of a car after a few years. Your body is yours for a lifetime.

What you don't know *can* hurt you. When considering cosmetic surgery, your best bet is to spend at least the same amount of time evaluating your surgery options as you would selecting your car.

Did You Know?

"I don't know where to start." "I'm just overwhelmed." "How do I get through the maze of information?" Comments like these show that quite often, much of the concern surrounding a cosmetic surgery decision is fear of the unknown. Studies support a direct correlation between informed patients, faster recoveries, and better outcomes. We all fear the unknown. This fear can cause stress, which is not an ally in your decision-making or healing process. Do all you can to reduce stress.

For some reason, once patients decide that they are interested in cosmetic surgery, they generally behave in one of two ways. Either they rush to make a decision, as if face-lifts were only available tomorrow and they have to decide today, or they become paralyzed with fear. Consider a healthy middle ground. Select a date several months away, or a season that works best with your schedule. Commit to doing three tasks per week that will implement your decision and increase your knowledge. (See "Informed Consent" on page 19.) The goal is to reduce your stress, increase your confidence, and do everything you can to produce safe, positive outcomes.

Part 1

The Cosmetic Surgery Decision

Part 1 is designed to lead you through the process of screening doctors and selecting the right doctor for you, emphasizing the importance of clear communication between you and your surgeon. The topic of fees and payment options for cosmetic surgery is also addressed. In addition, we present an overview of what you can expect during the pre- and postoperative periods, as well as general skin care guidelines. Finally, a compilation of advice from patients who have had cosmetic surgery provides a wealth of information from varied perspectives.

Remember that the more informed and prepared you are for the procedure you choose, the better your experience will be.

CHAPTER 1

You've Thought about It, but Where Do You Begin?

Why We Seek Cosmetic Surgery

Over the last several years, the number of cosmetic surgical procedures performed has steadily increased. According to the American Academy of Cosmetic Surgery (AACS), between 1996 and 1997 there was an average 40 percent increase in the top four cosmetic surgical procedures—liposuction, breast augmentation, eyelid surgery, and face-lift. That translates into 2.2 million Americans undergoing some form of cosmetic procedure in 1997. These numbers are expected to increase even more in each successive year.

Why are so many people choosing cosmetic surgery? The baby boomers of today no longer think or look like their mothers and fathers did when they were in their forties and fifties. Today's baby boomers also are more active and have more disposable income. Additionally, medical advances and technologies have become widely available and lower in price. As a result, cosmetic enhancements are no longer strictly reserved for the rich and famous.

OUR MOTIVATIONS

Motivations for having surgery vary by individual and gender. Some of the most common reasons for undergoing a cosmetic surgery procedure include the following:

- to look as young as one feels

- to correct asymmetry of a body part

- to get a psychological boost after a lifestyle change, such as divorce or pregnancy
- to maintain a youthful, vibrant appearance to effectively compete in the workplace

The way you look has a tremendous effect on the way you feel. The way you feel translates into the way you carry yourself and, therefore, the way others perceive you. We all understand the notion of a "bad hair day," which may dictate the way we feel and act for a short period of time.

As a society, we feel comfortable about driving expensive cars, decorating our homes, or adorning our bodies with jewelry. We are naturally concerned about our personal appearance. Cosmetic surgery does not have to be construed as self-indulgent. Contrary to some beliefs, people undergoing cosmetic surgery are not vain and narcissistic. Those who are seeking aesthetic changes are ordinary people who have areas on the face or body that can be improved or enhanced.

Naomi Wolf's book *The Beauty Myth* discusses, among other ideas, the politics of beauty, especially as it relates to women. She takes a historical, political, and perhaps, feminist perspective. She raises awareness of some of the more unrealistic expectations about beauty in our culture. She says, "Women today have more money, power, scope, and recognition than we've ever had before, but in terms of how we feel about ourselves physically, we may be no better off than our unliberated grandmothers."[1] Although this is not true for all of us, it does remind us of the need to be aware of our motivations for seeking surgery.

There is no doubt that everyone is conscious about his or her body image. These feelings are beginning to affect men, who now account for 25 percent of all cosmetic surgery patients. Years ago, early studies labeled those who wished to pursue cosmetic surgery as neurotic. Cosmetic surgery is now considered almost routine and certainly acceptable. The motivations for cosmetic surgery are very personal and are best described as being on a continuum, as illustrated on the next page. These motivations are neither good or bad nor right or wrong but should be observed in order to fully understand and be prepared for the process of a cosmetic surgery decision.

---

[1] Naomi Wolf, *The Beauty Myth*, (New York: William Morrow, 1991).

THE MOTIVATION CONTINUUM

When our motivations fall more onto the "typical" side of the continuum, we find that our expectations and the results are more closely aligned. Studies show that the outcome and perception of surgery are generally more positive. Studies have also shown that when our motivations fall on the "atypical" end of the continuum, greater levels of disappointment, dissatisfaction, and negative feelings about the surgical process are more likely to occur. An example of the Motivation Continuum is as follows:

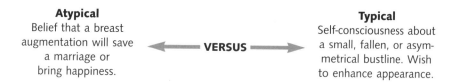

| **Atypical** | | **Typical** |
| Belief that a breast augmentation will save a marriage or bring happiness. | **← VERSUS →** | Self-consciousness about a small, fallen, or asymmetrical bustline. Wish to enhance appearance. |

Being honest and aware of our motivations is one of the factors determining our perception of the cosmetic surgery experience. It may mean the difference between "one of the best decisions I've ever made" and " I would never go through that again."

If you have any anxiety or doubt about your motivations for surgery, speak with a counselor. It is important to rule out any conditions that might be more psychological than physical, such as eating disorders, body dysmorphic disorder (BDD), or other related issues. For most of us, our motivations are healthy and not cause for worry, but no harm can come from examining your motivations.

If your motivations do not appear to fall into the extremely atypical area, cosmetic surgery could be the answer to what you may feel has detracted from your appearance in some way. It is an exciting decision and has some of the greatest rewards if approached wisely and with insight.

Cosmetic versus Reconstructive Surgery

Plastic surgery can be classified as reconstructive or cosmetic. As defined by the *Merriam-Webster Dictionary, reconstructive* "relates to the action of reconstructing, to rebuild"; *cosmetic* is "relating to beautifying the physical appearance."

RECONSTRUCTIVE PLASTIC SURGERY

Reconstructive surgery corrects and/or restores function and form to abnormalities or deformities that may be the result of a birth defect, accident, or disease. Examples of reconstructive plastic surgery are cleft lip repair, skin grafts to repair damaged skin, and breast reconstruction.

COSMETIC OR AESTHETIC PLASTIC SURGERY

Cosmetic surgery is performed to enhance, reshape, or improve one's appearance. The cosmetic patient usually falls within one of two groups. The first category is the patient who is interested in turning back the hands of time—generally on an aging face. The second category is usually made up of younger patients who have a feature (such as large breasts or a large nose) they feel is not in balance with the rest of their body and that may be affecting their self-image.

The term "plastic surgery" encompasses both reconstructive and cosmetic surgery, whereas "cosmetic surgery" generally refers only to aesthetic changes.

The Best and Worst Candidates for Cosmetic Surgery

Each year, millions of people choose to have aesthetic surgery to change the way they look. Some have noticeable changes, others subtle refinements. How can you tell if you should consider this option?

BEST CANDIDATES FOR COSMETIC SURGERY

Ideal cosmetic surgery candidates should

- recognize a specific area of their body or face that could be improved

- have a strong personal desire to make a change

- be aware of, and honest about, their motivations for having the surgery

- realize that plastic surgery can only change how they look and feel to a certain extent (it is not a guarantee of happiness or better relationships)

- have realistic expectations not only concerning the outcome but also regarding the necessary preparations, the actual surgery, the recovery period, and the discomfort

- be willing to modify their lifestyle during recovery, e.g., by stopping smoking or avoiding alcohol and restricting movements and exercise

- have a willingness to comply with the physician's pre- and postoperative instructions

- understand the risks and complications of the procedure(s) they are considering

WORST CANDIDATES FOR COSMETIC SURGERY

In contrast, the worst candidates for cosmetic surgery include

- anyone assuming that surgery will bring perfection

- anyone overly obsessive about a small deficit

- those undergoing surgery to please someone else

- those who make a hasty decision to undergo surgery immediately

- anyone suffering or emerging from a traumatic or emotionally tumultuous event

- anyone with psychological symptoms or disorders including, but not limited to, paranoia, depression, narcissism, body dysmorphic disorder, anorexia, or bulimia

- anyone experiencing hormone swings or who has recently begun treatment to stabilize hormonal imbalances

- those with untreated thyroid disorders

- anyone with a bleeding disorder, such as hemophilia

- pregnant or lactating women

- drug or alcohol abusers

- those with autoimmune system disorders or deficiencies

- smokers

Being honest with yourself and your doctor about any of the above that would make you an unfavorable candidate for surgery could save your life. When contemplating aesthetic changes, a tendency to overlook certain medical or mental healthcare conditions is great, because we are focused on the outcome, not the process. But it is the process that gets us where we want to go. Using a golf swing as an example—certainly, you must line up your shot (longer range planning), but you must focus on the elements that make up your swing, and most of all, keep your eye on the ball (doing the task at hand)—only then will you reach your goal of a safe, positive result.

Men and Cosmetic Surgery

Today, more men than ever before are seeking cosmetic surgery. National statistics indicate that approximately 25 percent of cosmetic surgery patients are men.

There are several reasons for the upswing in men having cosmetic surgery:

- competition and a perceived focus on youth in the business world
- the increased awareness and acceptance of cosmetic surgery by society in general
- men taking a more active role in their healthcare decisions

Men make these types of decisions differently than women. Women may talk for years about having surgery and generally take a lot longer to decide. Men, however, don't talk about surgery as much—but they are thinking about it. For example, it is highly unlikely that a conversation between two male friends at a baseball game would ever turn to the subject of face-lifts, whereas in an all-female outing, the subject frequently comes up for discussion.

Additionally, when men consider cosmetic surgery, they tend to be more proactive in seeking information than women and then act on their decision(s) more quickly. In contrast, statistics show that men are less compliant with follow-up care and instructions and tend to be less satisfied with their results than women.

What procedures are men having most frequently? The following is a partial list:

- blepharoplasty (eyelid surgery)
- face-lift
- brow lift
- liposuction
- hair restoration

- abdominoplasty (tummy tuck)
- male breast reduction
- rhinoplasty (nose reshaping)
- penile enhancement
- otoplasty (ear pinning)

In most cases, the procedures for men are the same as for women, with a few modifications. For instance, in facial surgery the incision sites may be different. A man's hairline is taken into consideration to allow for sideburns and the potential for baldness or thinning hair. In addition, men tend to have thicker skin than women. This is one reason why men seem to age more gracefully than women. Thicker skin does not wrinkle as easily and generally does not turn into looser "crepey" skin, but rather will form into deeper folds.

Healing may differ because a man's facial area usually contains hair, which means the blood supply is greater. This could result in a greater risk of bleeding. However, the increased blood supply may also facilitate healing.

What If Those around You Are Not Supportive?

Be aware that, for many different reasons, your spouse, significant other, or other family members may not be supportive of your decision. Why do loved ones act this way? Some reasons may be

- they love you because of who you are, not how you look
- they fear that you will not be the same person after the surgery
- you may seem to lose your ethnicity
- they may view the "new you" as a possible threat to the relationship. If you change, will the relationship also change?
- they may have an aversion to anything "surgical"
- you may seem vain or selfish to them
- they may object to the amount of money the surgery will cost
- they may feel unwilling, unable, or inadequate to cope with the household situation while you are recuperating

If the lack of support will interfere with your recovery—i.e., cooking dinner, cleaning house, childcare, stress—you may want to postpone your decision or seek support elsewhere. As an option, you may wish to contract for household assistance during your recovery.

Friends and family can help by listening and reacting nonjudgmentally to their loved one. Theoretically and legally, an adult who is mentally competent has the right to pursue a surgical decision. Patients, however, recover more quickly when they have support from those who care. For family or other emotional problems, you may want to seek professional advice.

CHAPTER 2

Selecting a Doctor

Informed Consent

Informed decision making is the precursor to informed consent. Informed consent means we understand something before we agree to it. In order to be fully prepared, we need information on which to base our decision to proceed.

ACTIVE RESPONSIBILITY

Legally and ethically, doctors must disclose risks as well as benefits or anticipated improvements to the prospective patient. Although a patient signs an informed consent form before surgery, just how informed are these patients? The consent forms you are asked to sign are written and provided by either the physician's attorney or the doctor himself. The form, therefore, is designed to protect the doctor—not you—in the event of a complication. If you are looking for someone to blame (the physician) if a complication occurs, then sign the consent form on the dotted line. Conversely, if you are seeking the avoidance of risk, then do your homework. Once you have taken *personal responsibility* to do your own research, you can and should feel comfortable signing those forms (if you agree with the contents and spirit of the document).

Becoming informed can be an adventure, should you choose to view it that way. Although it takes time and commitment, it is incredibly exciting to seek out the information that will contribute to your successful outcome. The amount of research will vary from person to person according to time and energy available. Nonetheless, taking responsibility minimally requires the following:

Do Not Be Hasty in Your Decision

It is difficult to keep up with the advances in the field of cosmetic surgery. Numerous publications, books, and Internet resources are available for you to compare the many factors involved in cosmetic surgery. You may find that the latest technology is not the best for you. As difficult as this may be—*wait*. Wait until you've thoroughly investigated the available information before you schedule appointments or choose a doctor.

Allow yourself some time for research and to become prepared for your cosmetic surgery decision. Pick a date three months in the future as the target date to begin your physician consultations. During that time, make a commitment to read a book every two weeks, investigate several Internet sites per week, and let the information wash over you. You'll soak up more than you realize, and since you have been so well prepared, you will be much more comfortable with your physician-selection process and the surgeon you ultimately choose to perform your procedure.

Have a Doctor Selection Plan

In order to successfully choose surgeons to visit, you must narrow your choices. If you do not have a selection plan, all the information you've gathered is still valuable, but you could waste a lot of time with doctors who are not suited to you. Since you now have a good deal of information from reading, visiting Internet sites, and listening to others' experiences, use that to carefully select the doctors with whom you will be spending *your* valuable time.

Begin with recommendations from friends, look at local articles written about surgeons in your area, and watch for radio or television news stories featuring plastic or cosmetic surgeons. See which names are mentioned most often in a favorable way. These names should correspond with the procedures you are considering. For example, if you are interested in a face-lift, and the doctors that you hear about most often have great results with liposuction, these doctors may not necessarily be the best suited to you.

Once you have gathered at least three doctors' names, you can begin to conduct telephone interviews with the staff at their offices. Your phone interviews with the doctor's staff should include asking questions about the doctor's qualifications, his experience with your particular procedure, whether the staff has undergone or would undergo surgery with the doctor for whom they work, and what services the office offers to patients.

Shop Around Carefully

See more than one doctor, no matter how much you like the first one. Marked differences exist between doctors' techniques, approaches, and comfort levels with various procedures. Remember—when you visit surgeons or other doctors, they are marketing the procedures and techniques in which *they* are experienced. They may not discuss other options that may be available to you if they do not perform them. That does not necessarily make them bad doctors or even guilty of withholding information. After all, if you go to a Toyota dealer and ask which kind of car is best for you, what do you think the response will be?

From a purely business perspective, why should the doctor be obligated to tell you about procedures he *does not* perform? The onus is on you to find out what is available and then question the doctors as to the appropriateness of that option for you. After discussing all the options, *you*—along with your chosen doctor—should make an informed decision.

Now that you have become educated about all of your options and you've followed a plan, trust your judgment. If all of the doctors seem knowledgeable, skilled, and experienced, select the one who listens best, has the most compassion, loves what he does, and whom you admire. These factors should be the "tie-breaker," if you find yourself in a position where a choice is difficult.

Don't Be Emotional

Emotions can sometimes lead to making a hasty cosmetic surgery decision based on an advertisement or a loved one's suggestions. It is wonderful to dream, but unrealistic or hasty decisions can turn that dream into a nightmare. Asking for assistance from former patients who have had positive *and* negative results will help to ground your expectations and dreams in reality.

Know Your Goals

The goal of surgery is improvement, not perfection. Knowing this will take the pressure off both you and your physician. It is imperative that you share your goals and motivations so that your doctor understands what you are looking for. This lays the groundwork for open communication and helps to dispel any misunderstandings before they take hold.

One of the most exciting technologies available in the cosmetic surgery industry is computer imaging. If you have access to computer imaging (see the

"Computer Imaging" section on page 38) either through a cosmetic surgery consulting firm or other facility, it can be a wonderful tool to help you visualize the possibilities before visiting your doctor. It can also help to minimize presurgery stress. If you do not have access to computer imaging, consider gathering some photographs that display in an unfavorable manner the feature you wish to change. Make two copies and draw with pens or markers on one copy. Slenderize your legs, take a bump out of your nose, or reduce your tummy. Your drawings or a computer image is only a rendition and not necessarily clinically achievable, but it can start you thinking about and communicating the kinds of changes you'd like to see.

Recognize the Limitations of Informed Consent

Keep in mind that true informed consent is always difficult for numerous reasons. For example:

- Doctors attempt to, but can't always, convey all matters involved with the surgery decision. Whether because of time or the sheer volume of material that could be discussed, not all information gets relayed.

- Patients often have selective hearing. They may ignore what they don't want to hear.

- Statistically, few doctors have experienced cosmetic surgery themselves.

- The doctors' perception, generally, is that upon *completion* of the surgery, the greatest percentage of their work is concluded; whereas the patient's perception is that care continues *after* surgery.

- Doctors tend to focus on the clinical or technical aspects of care and less on the emotional/psychological aspects. Aesthetic surgery patients (unlike those with reconstructive or functional problems) are almost always motivated by emotional concerns.

- Patients aren't always interested in hearing about risks or complications for fear it might steer them away from a decision that may have been difficult in the first place.

Use a Consulting Firm

One alternative is to use a consulting firm to help you wade through the myriad of options. But here, too, you must choose carefully. Not all consulting firms are alike. Choose one with a comfortable environment where you do not feel rushed. Consulting fees vary based on the services available. These are essential features to look for in a consulting group:

- The firm's expertise lies in *more* than just the "patient experience." The consultants are trained and are overseen by a surgeon or medical advisory committee to assure that information given out by the consultants is accurate, timely, and topical.

- Your consultant has had cosmetic surgery.

- The firm uses a formal screening and credentialing process for doctors that includes verification of malpractice history and an inquiry to the National Practitioner Data Bank, at the very least. Credentialing in accordance with the National Committee for Quality Assurance (NCQA) is preferred. (See "Physician Screening and Selection" on page 26.)

- Referrals to more than one doctor are provided—preferably to two to three doctors.

- Referrals are only given to physicians who agree to operate out of an accredited surgical center. (See "Surgical Facility Accreditation" on page 32.)

- Ongoing support and research are provided.

- Computer imaging is available. (This feature is helpful, but not necessary.)

Ensure Clear Communication

As you can see, the potential for miscommunication is great. At the very least, listening carefully, asking questions, and achieving agreement on issues to be included on your consent forms will create an open and communicative environment. This will go a long way in fostering a positive patient-physician relationship.

Specialty Groups within Cosmetic Surgery

The politics or economics in any field can explain a lot. It is no different within the field of plastic and cosmetic surgery. Recent changes in our healthcare system have been devastating to some physicians, while others have thrived and embraced the environment of change. Either way, the practice of medicine is very different from what it was even five to ten years ago. Because of the increased competition among doctors, standards that used to be regarded as sacred in the medical domain—such as respect, creating a unified front on issues, and not speaking poorly of other medical professionals—have relaxed quite a bit. Some good and not-so-good has come of this.

One good result of these changes is the breaking of the silence that once protected a colleague when the quality of care or public safety was at risk. As long as proper legal and ethical standards are adhered to, we must continue to support those who report incompetence, impairment, or criminal activity by their fellow doctors.

On the other hand, we all lose when doctors speak poorly of their colleagues as a result of fear, economics, or the desire to keep others out of a particular "club." Some physician specialty groups feel they are the only ones qualified to perform certain procedures. As a result, major legal battles have been fought among these groups with very little effect on the end users—the public. Ultimately, the public is concerned about the surgeons' skill, training, and experience in the specialty or the procedures they perform. When professionals voluntarily separate themselves, we lose collaborative efforts that could benefit us all.

This kind of behavior is inappropriate and unprofessional. When questioned closely about this problem, some doctors admit that exclusionary tactics are more the result of personality conflicts than any lack of expertise. Many different specialties have contributed much to the techniques and technology used today in the cosmetic surgery field. If you encounter exaggerated claims from a cosmetic surgeon, understand the reasons for them, but you may consider looking for someone who isn't so threatened.

The physician you choose to perform your body procedure may not necessarily be best suited for your facial procedure. If you are considering liposuction and a face-lift, do not feel pressured to have them both performed by the same physician simply because it seems to be easier or less expensive. If your choice of physician for your facial procedure is different (for whatever reason), inquire if the two physicians are willing to perform surgery in a cooperative manner. If not, consider having one of the procedures at another time. Remember—this is your body, your face, and your choice.

An umbrella organization known as the American Board of Medical Specialties (ABMS) recognizes only those physicians who are board certified by one of its member boards. A "board" is an organization made up of physicians (whether recognized by ABMS or not) who have created educational and practice standards to which each of its member physicians must adhere to be viewed as competent in a particular specialty. This recognition indicates that the physician has completed many hours of training in the specialty and has shown competency through written and oral examination.

Some boards are not recognized by ABMS. The reasons for this are varied. Certain physicians believe ABMS decisions are politically motivated. In their opinion, ABMS has refused membership to boards that compete with existing boards. For example, one physician pointed out that podiatry is not a recognized specialty because it competes with orthopedics.

The field of cosmetic surgery has become highly competitive. When competition increases, we often see an increase in animosity between the competing parties. The animosity between several specialty groups within cosmetic surgery has grown to the point where lawsuits have been fought over specialty board recognition and which board's qualifications are superior. Sadly, much of the conflict seems in vain, as it has not served to increase the quality of medical care. The real loss is the lack of cooperation that could be of value for the ultimate end user—the patient. Should you ever encounter a doctor who speaks poorly about another doctor, or a specialty in general, you may want to assess whether he is the best choice. It is wise to keep discussions with a doctor focused on what a doctor can do for you, *not* on the shortcomings of another doctor or specialty.

The general population is not concerned with the political wrangling of doctors and their world. Of course, they do want to make sure that there are some standards to which doctors must be held. The individual credentials of your physician should be evaluated for skill, training, experience, and positive results. As we have mentioned earlier, board certification does not necessarily indicate that you have chosen a "good doctor." Depending on the procedure (facial or body), you will be well served to select a doctor who is board certified by either the American Board of Plastic Surgery or the American Board of Facial Plastic and Reconstructive Surgery as a starting point.

The following are some of the common specialties (already discussed) and additional specialties represented in the cosmetic surgery field today:

PLASTIC AND RECONSTRUCTIVE SURGEONS

These doctors are certified by the American Board of Plastic Surgery (ABMS Member Board) and trained in both body and facial procedures.

FACIAL PLASTIC SURGEONS

These doctors are certified by the American Board of Facial Plastic and Reconstructive Surgery, usually trained in otolaryngology/ENT (ear, nose and throat) and certified by the American Board of Otolaryngology (ABMS Member Board), and trained in procedures of the face, head, and neck only.

COSMETIC DERMATOLOGISTS

These doctors are certified by the American Board of Dermatology (ABMS Member Board) and trained in the treatment of diseases of the skin and often in laser procedures, liposuction, hair removal, and other procedures.

OCCULOPLASTIC SURGEONS

Certified by the American Board of Ophthalmology (ABMS Member Board) and trained in disease, sickness, or injury to the eyes and often in eyelid surgery, laser surgery, and other procedures.

Physician Screening and Selection

Many questions are asked about cosmetic surgery. It seems to be a subject that fascinates us all, whether we are personally interested or not. But the number one question, far exceeding all others, is "How do I find a qualified surgeon?" It is odd that we don't ask the same question or spend as much time planning for a gallbladder operation or knee surgery. In addition, we seem better able to accept the sad occasions when tragedies result from such non-elective surgeries. When we hear of a tragic outcome resulting from cosmetic surgery, on the other hand, the public outcry seems greater. Also, a subtle sort of blame (often, not so subtle) is placed on the patient, as if she somehow contributed to her own tragedy, merely by wanting to look better and subjecting herself to unnecessary surgery. While it is a scary prospect to undergo cosmetic surgery and risk emerging with a disfigurement or worse, most people are concerned about a less-than-desired result—that their expectations will not be met.

How can we minimize the risks? It all begins with how you select your surgeon. The top three sources patients generally use to find their surgeons are as follows:

1. **The Yellow Pages**—The telephone book can be a great source of information, but what do the ads tell you about a physician's qualifications? The bigger the city, the more overwhelming this method of searching is.

2. **Local magazines**—If you read an article written about a particular doctor in a magazine, be aware that many publications will only print articles about physicians who advertise with them. There is nothing wrong with this arrangement; however, it can give you a biased view of a doctor's abilities.

3. **A referral from someone you know**—This is probably the best option. Remember that although your friend may have had a great face-lift, her doctor may not be the best doctor to choose for a breast augmentation or liposuction.

THE CREDENTIALING PROCESS

A credentialing or screening process is an equitable method of determining a physician's qualifications. The cosmetic surgery industry is growing quickly, and doctors are attracted to it in large numbers, partly because of managed care and its fee arrangements with physicians. Currently, no formal guidelines exist for cosmetic surgeons. This chapter outlines the standards that should be implemented as a basis for measuring quality and ultimately for a full-fledged quality management program. A formal credentialing process would help to guard against any doctor without adequate training or experience offering aesthetic surgery services. Some consulting and referral companies are in the beginning stages of developing such a program, but more needs to be accomplished in this segment of healthcare.

The managed care industry uses as one of its screening standards the National Committee for Quality Assurance (NCQA) guidelines. NCQA is an accreditation entity that applies quality measurement protocols to determine if physicians meet certain quality standards. NCQA addresses physicians in general, not cosmetic surgeons specifically, so additional criteria must be applied to plastic/cosmetic surgeons. A comprehensive physician-screening process can provide the methodology for finding a talented and competent surgeon.

USING A CONSULTING AND REFERRAL COMPANY

By using an information and referral company, you do not have to do the "leg-work" of collecting, investigating, and verifying physicians' credentials on your own. In addition, as an individual rather than a healthcare company, in some instances you will not have access to all the information that a referral company has access to. You are paying a referral or consulting fee for convenience and peace of mind. Also, the firm's services can direct you to surgeons who have already gone through the credentialing process and to whom you can immediately go for your physician consultations.

Since the credentialing process can take up to several months, you cannot bring a physician's name to the firm and ask whether you should visit him. You can, however, make a suggestion about a surgeon you have heard of and request that the referral company contact him to see if he would consider participation. At that time, the referral company would either meet with him or send out an application for participation. As information services increase in speed, you may in the near future be able to suggest a name and have the physician's qualifications verified in a shorter period of time. Most likely this would require an additional fee but could be worth it.

Please note that a doctor may choose *not* to participate in a referral company for many reasons. A doctor may be older, nearing retirement, and not wish to see new patients. Some doctors see a referral company as a form of advertising and are philosophically against advertising. Other physicians may be in a geographically desirable area and feel that they are growing their practices without any outside help. A doctor's choice to participate does not indicate whether he is a good or bad doctor. That is something only a thorough and fair credentialing process can reveal.

Physician selection through credentialing is probably the single most important and complex function that the referral organization should handle for you. When a physician is interested in becoming a part of a referral panel, the process should begin with a formal application for participation provided by the referral company.

The company should investigate and verify all of the information collected. An internal credentialing committee made up of several physicians and staff from the organization should convene upon receipt of a completed application to check it for accuracy and completeness and assess any areas that may require additional input from the applicant. The application could also be sent to an independent credentialing verification organization (CVO), which performs the due diligence necessary to substantiate the physician's statements. A comprehensive packet containing validation of all data, including letters from the educational institution, hospital(s), and malpractice insurance company should be kept on file for each doctor. All of this information combined with other criteria allows the referral company to profile the practice and the status of the physician who is applying. Once this information has been returned and verified, if it meets or exceeds the credentialing standards and the doctor has complied with any other requests, he should be accepted onto the physician referral panel.

There should be no obligation for you to use the panel doctors. However, physicians have often agreed to waive their normal consultation charges for patients who use the services of the referral company. This can actually result in savings, since physician consultation fees can range from $75 to $175. If you are referred to two to three physicians, as you should be, you can make up the cost of the visit to the consultant. Doctors make this offer because they feel reputable information-and-referral companies can make their job easier—a well-informed patient may be more likely to proceed with surgery and is much better prepared. This is good for the doctor and good for the patient.

CREDENTIALING CRITERIA

The data listed on the next two pages indicates the kinds of information you will want to know about your chosen surgeon. If you are using a consulting firm, you should ask if this information is requested from the physicians and then submitted in full for panel consideration.

If you are doing research on your own, the following charts describe the data collected in detail and why it is gathered. This should act as a guideline so that you can collect as many of these items as possible. (See "Taking Control" on page 35 and "Resources" on page 273.)

DATA AVAILABLE TO INDIVIDUALS

As an individual, versus a healthcare entity, you will find some areas in which access to information is blocked. Unfortunately, it will probably be some time before the general public will be able to gain access to more information about

SAMPLE OF NCQA CRITERIA

CRITERIA	DATA COLLECTED	WHY?
Provider identification	Demographic information: addresses (past and present), Social Security numbers, tax identification numbers	To make certain that this doctor is who he says he is
Malpractice carrier information	Name of insurance company, policy number, coverage limits, dates the policy is in effect	To verify adequate levels of coverage to meet requirements, and any lapses or terminations of coverage
Malpractice history	Any past or pending claims or judgments and detailed disclosure of event(s)	To ascertain the history, if any, and extent of the doctor's involvement in malpractice claims
Professional status	Degree, specialty, board certification, and advertised practice specialty	For verification of board certification and experience in specialty
Education and work history	Schooling, graduation dates, lapses in education, internship, residency, and fellowship start and end dates, and five-year work history	For verification
Hospital affiliations	Type of affiliation (full or courtesy) and any positions held	To verify that physician is in good standing
Licensing and registrations	State medical license, DEA, Medicare/Medicaid information	To become apprised of any limitations or disciplinary actions that might render a doctor unqualified
Provider questionnaire	Answers to questions about organizational suspensions, revocations, or limitations as well as criminal, mental health, substance abuse, and sexual deviancy history and physical limitations or impairments	To attain the highest possible safety standards because patients are often in vulnerable positions in a surgical setting
Attestation to truthfulness	Signature guaranteeing truthfulness	To further confirm physician's honesty and provide greater access to recourse, if required
NPDB query	Current data from the National Practitioner Data Bank, which reports sanctions, revocations, and limitations on licenses; information about any changes in the status of a license or disciplinary action should be received frequently (re-credentialing) and updated immediately	Another way to assure the reliability of information gathered and an unbiased source for this information; unfortunately, this information is currently available to healthcare entities only

CRITERIA SPECIFIC TO PLASTIC/COSMETIC SURGERY

CRITERIA	DATA COLLECTED	WHY?
Frequency of procedures	How often procedures are performed, number of consultations/conversions to surgery, rejection rate for surgery, experience with ethnic populations, age/sex mix of patients	To ascertain the doctor's experience
Patient services	"On-call" arrangements, patient advocacy, skin care services, postoperative gifts, and so on	To ascertain what services are rendered and what differentiates this office
Surgical location and accreditation	Location at which the doctor most frequently operates—a public outpatient or the doctor's own surgical facility. If owned by the surgeon, is the facility accredited by AAAAHC, AAAHC, or JCAHO (see "Surgical Facility Accreditation" on page 32). Type of anesthesia services available; whether M.D. or nurse anesthetists are on staff or contracted	To ascertain the safety and quality standards of the facility in which the doctor operates
Professional affiliations	Membership in societies and organizations	To verify affiliations and the doctor's standing within the organization
Fee schedule	Surgical fees for procedures; facility charges are reported as a range, as these fees vary based on the procedure performed and time needed	To compare fee ranges for several physicians at once and for patient/client convenience
Patient references	Interviews of former patients	To evaluate patient reactions, satisfaction, and experience
Professional references	Interviews of colleagues	To gain knowledge of colleagues' opinions
Site visits	Evaluation of cleanliness, patient confidentiality, staff knowledge and courtesy, efficiency, access, and so on	To assess whether the office is a comfortable environment for patients
Observing surgery	Observation of how surgeons conduct themselves in their environment	To observe interaction between physician, staff, and patient
Before and after photographs	Approximately six to eight patient photographs	Evidence of work

a physician. However, the good news is that you can take some actions on your own. The chart on the next page outlines the levels of access you may have regarding certain criteria. The rules in your state may vary, but use this chart as a guide. It is imperative that you gather and evaluate all the information that is available to you. (See "Resources" on page 273.)

Surgical Facility Accreditation

Many more surgeons than ever before are building their own surgical centers or operating rooms in which to perform surgery. This allows physicians to have greater control over staffing, scheduling, procedures, and supplies. Having procedures performed in a physician's surgical facility is usually less expensive than surgery done in the hospital or public outpatient setting. Fees for cosmetic surgery are usually broken down into several different components: the surgical fee and facility fees for the cost of the operating room, supplies, and sometimes anesthesia. (See "Cosmetic Surgery Fees" on page 43.) When a physician owns his operating room he can retain the facility fees that would normally go to the hospital or outpatient facility.

While hospitals and outpatient clinics have generally met the highest levels of accreditation, individually owned surgical suites can opt out of some levels of accreditation. Centers wishing to be approved for Medicare reimbursement must undergo a site inspection. At this time, approximately 90 percent of surgery centers are Medicare approved. At the state level, forty-one states currently require inspections before a surgery center may be opened for business. State officials or their delegates perform these evaluations.

The next level of accreditation is a voluntary process performed by an organization or agency other than a governmental institution to assess and measure the quality of services rendered in a particular healthcare setting. The evaluation of quality involves self-assessment and adherence to the standards created by the accrediting body, whose members are practicing healthcare professionals. After a thorough review, accreditation is granted once it is determined that compliance with these standards has been met. Often, accreditation can be awarded on a provisional basis for six months to a year if it is deemed that there is substantial compliance but that continued compliance cannot be clearly demonstrated at the time of the review.

ACCESSIBILITY OF DATA TO INDIVIDUALS

CRITERIA	ACCESS
Provider information	No
Malpractice information	No
Malpractice history	No
Professional status	It is possible that this information will be released to you; some organizations may only release this data with an authorization from the physician and may charge an administration fee
Education	Yes; fee could be charged
Hospital affiliation	Yes; fee could be charged
Licensing and registration	It is possible that this information will be released to you; some organizations may only release this data with an authorization from the physician and may charge an administration fee.
Provider questionnaire	No
Provider attestation of truthfulness	No
National Practitioner Data Bank (NPDB)	No
Frequency of procedures	Yes
Patient services	Yes
Surgical location— Accreditation	The physician may or may not provide access voluntarily; an accreditation entity may reveal the status but could charge an administration fee; ask to see certification
Professional affiliations	Yes
Fee schedule guaranteed for a period of time	Some physicians will guarantee their fees for a period of time— usually three months from the time of the physician's consultation
Patient references	Yes
Professional references	It is possible that this information will be released to you; some physicians may speak with you only after authorization from the chosen doctor
Site visits	The doctor may offer prospective patients the opportunity to view the offices and surgical facility; in most instances an in-depth evaluation of office procedures that relate to OSHA compliance or medical/surgical regulations will not be allowed
Observing surgery	No
Before and after pictures	Yes

A physician's decision to proceed with voluntary accreditation is a sign that he has the ultimate safety and welfare of patients in mind. The willingness to undergo evaluation confirms that interest because accreditation standards are high. The following are just a few of the criteria necessary to receive and maintain accreditation:

- appropriately trained personnel assisting in the provision of surgical services
- life-support and monitoring equipment
- resuscitation equipment
- an anesthesiologist or nurse anesthetist present during surgical procedures
- operating room designed and equipped so that surgery can be performed in a safe manner
- emergency procedures detailed in writing

You may want to contact an accrediting organization (see "Resources" on page 273) to find out if the doctor you have chosen operates in an accredited facility. Your own credentialing strategy, or that of a consulting firm you use, ought to require accreditation of the surgeon's own facility or an agreement to operate out of one that is certified.

CHAPTER 3

Meeting Your Doctor

Taking Control

Feeling in control can make a big difference when making a cosmetic surgery decision. Just reading and learning more about procedures can alert you to the various options a doctor may present, directing you to find someone who specializes in the procedure you are contemplating. It can make a difference in your recovery because you know what to expect and are less anxious. Even if as an individual you won't have access to all the data that healthcare entities do, you can still do a lot on your own to take control. It is your body and your life. Taking any one of the following actions will greatly increase your chances of a successful result. The more you research, the better your ultimate decision will be.

FOLLOW THROUGH ON AVAILABLE INFORMATION

If you are going to do your own legwork, make sure you gather all the information that is available to you (see "Resources" on page 273). Often, if a prospective patient likes a particular doctor, she may stop trying to verify his credentials. An element of trust is essential, but verifying that trust could save your life.

CALL YOUR STATE MEDICAL LICENSING BOARD

Although some states won't give out a lot of information, they'll usually tell you whether the doctor is licensed to practice in the state. This is basic information, but don't fail to ask this simple question. Just because a doctor has offices and staff does not mean he automatically has a license to practice.

VISIT A SURGEON'S OFFICE BEFORE YOU MAKE AN APPOINTMENT

Often, we know right away when we walk into a room, house, or office whether we are comfortable. Although this approach is very subjective and no indication of the surgeon's talents, it is a way to narrow your search from the overwhelming number of physician choices. Visit the office, let them know that you are considering scheduling a physician consultation, and ask if you can look around, meet a staff member or two, and just get a general feel for the environment. You can find out a lot—everything from cleanliness to staff friendliness and helpfulness. Notice whether the staff seems stressed or if patients seem to be waiting a long time, and how the staff interacts with the patients. All of this information can be valuable in your search.

USE A CONSULTING SERVICE

Considering what you get, the fee might just be worth it. With such a tremendous amount of information to research, it is sometimes difficult and time-consuming to get all of the answers you want. Using an information-and-referral service can be a good idea for several reasons:

- A referral service generally has access to all information and is not blocked from organizational health and reporting agencies.
- It's more convenient. Thorough physician screening and selection is an extremely long and tedious process.
- You won't be in an adversarial relationship with physicians. Asking questions is your right, but some questions are difficult to ask. When a third party asks the questions, *you* can concentrate on building a communicative relationship with your chosen doctor.
- Physician consultation fees could be waived, so you may save money.
- You'll benefit from the experience of the consultants and get the facts about recovery, procedures, and so on.

DON'T RUSH

Good decisions are rarely rushed into. Some factor is almost always left out as a result of a hasty decision.

READ

Knowledge is power. Many publications have been written about cosmetic surgery, both by patients and surgeons. The more you read, the more knowledgeable you are.

OBTAIN INDUSTRY PUBLICATIONS

You can subscribe to *Cosmetic Surgery Times* and *Dermatology Times,* as well as other publications, even if you are not a doctor. Use the publication names in a keyword search online to find ordering information.

INVESTIGATE INTERNET RESOURCES

Search under "Cosmetic Surgery/Plastic Surgery/Aesthetic Surgery," and you will be amazed at the information that you will find. Immerse yourself, visit many sites, and get a general feel for this industry.

PLAN

There is more to this process than you might think. It is real surgery. You would spend time planning if you were scheduled for any other surgery. Be as thorough planning for cosmetic surgery. Planning for your surgery also includes taking care of nonclinical tasks: making sure your house is in order, paying household bills in advance, and arranging for assistance with children and/or pets so you won't be saddled with chores during your recovery time. (See "Patient Tips and Secrets" on page 61.)

DON'T RULE OUT TRAVELING

If you find a doctor who is not in your local area, then traveling for your surgery could work well. You'll need to consider accommodations, additional costs, and follow-up care, but traveling is an option and may be worth it. Some individuals actually like the idea of going out of town and being away from their normal surroundings so they can concentrate on nothing but healing.

VISIT SEVERAL DOCTORS

Consult with at least three doctors, no matter how much you like one of them. Because the process of screening physicians can be intensive, you could have a tendency to schedule surgery with the first doctor who seems competent and likable. Resist that tendency because there may be better options available—and you can always come back to your first choice. Compare this to buying a house. You would never select one house without seeing all of your choices.

INTERVIEW FORMER PATIENTS

The physicians you visit should be able to give you names of former patients with whom to speak about their experiences. At the very least, the doctor should contact patients who would be willing to speak with you and arrange a mutually agreeable time to speak.

Ask former patients about good experiences, as well as situations that they wish had been handled differently. You might also wish to ask whether the patient is the doctor's close friend or family member before you begin discussions.

Computer Imaging

Computer or video imaging is an innovative way to answer the question, "I wonder what I'd look like after cosmetic surgery?" Using a camera and special computer software, your appearance can be altered on the screen right before your eyes so that you can better visualize the outcome of cosmetic surgery. Perhaps you aren't sure about having a procedure performed or you're considering multiple procedures. Computer imaging can assist with your decision. Many people use computer imaging as a way of minimizing any presurgery stress. It's a fun, fast, and effective way to explore the possibilities.

The images that will be produced for you are approximations, but they look remarkably close to actual results. And there's no safer, simpler way for you to objectively preview the procedure you are contemplating. Computer imaging involves you by giving you the opportunity to share what you like and dislike about your current features or a proposed change. Having a computer imaging session will allow you to better communicate your requested changes with your chosen doctor. The use of the computer image can help alleviate unrealistic self-images that a patient may harbor. It may also help you gain the support of family members and friends because they will be able to see the proposed changes beforehand.

Computer imaging is a powerful technology, and the goal is to provide you with a picture of a clinically achievable outcome. However, it is important to remember that it is a computer image only. You and your surgeon must discuss what is ultimately possible.

Physicians often feel strongly about computer imaging, whether they utilize this technology or not. Among those who do offer imaging, the general consensus is that it is an effective communication tool. Physicians who do not offer it usually cite encouraging unrealistic expectations as their reason.

This computer technology is relatively new so the choice of offering computer imaging is a business decision made individually by each practice. From a marketing perspective, some physicians often feel that they may be at a disadvantage if they do not offer it. Ultimately, it should not be viewed as criteria for physician selection.

Questions to Ask the Doctor

The goal of the physician consultation is to leave with more concrete information than, "I like this surgeon." Unless you write your questions or thoughts down and bring them with you, the likelihood that you'll forget something or never really get to the important points is high. Also, there is often a great deal of stress when we schedule appointments such as these, even when we're excited and looking forward to the results.

You are meeting your doctor for the first time. How can you make the most of your time with him? First, write a list of questions you have for the doctor and bring it with you to your appointment. Next, to make the meeting go more smoothly, do not bring your children to your appointment. Most physicians' offices do not have the staff to watch your children during your consultation with the doctor. You are making an important decision, and your undivided attention is essential to your health and well-being. Finally, and most important, if the doctor uses a term or phrase that you do not understand, have him explain it in words that you do understand.

The following are some important questions you may want to include in your list:

- What are your qualifications?
- How many times have you performed this procedure?

- What are the surgical risks?

- What kinds of complications could occur?

- Can I get the same results without surgery or with a less invasive option?

- How much will the operation cost?

- Does your fee include all of my preoperative and postoperative appointments?

- Will my insurance cover this surgery? If so, who files for reimbursement?

- Where will I have the surgery done? Are there choices?

- Is the surgical site accredited?

- Is monitoring and resuscitation equipment available on site?

- Are you ACLS (advanced cardiac life support) certified? Is your certification current?

- Will I be under local, IV (intravenous) sedation, or general anesthesia?

- Is there an anesthesiologist who is a medical doctor or is there a nurse anesthetist?

- How is the surgery performed?

- Where and how will the incisions be made?

- Are there any other surgical options or techniques available that *you* may or may not perform?

- What are the advantages/disadvantages of each of the options?

- Why do you feel that the approach you are recommending is the best one for me?

- How long will the surgery take?

- What kind of dressings will you apply and when will they be removed?

- Will there be any drains inserted, and how long will the drains be left in place?

- Will I have stitches? Are they dissolvable? If not, when will they be removed?

- Will I be able to go home directly after surgery?

- Will there be swelling? How long will it last?

- Will there be bruising? How long will it last?

- Am I supposed to apply cold compresses/ice packs to control swelling? How often?

- What kind of special garments, if any, will I be required to wear and for how long? Where can I purchase them?

- Do I have to sleep in any special position?

- How much discomfort can I expect?

- Are you (the doctor) going to be in town during the critical postoperative period (the first week)? If not, who covers for you when you are not available?

- Are you (the doctor) available to call if I have any questions during my recovery? Is there a staff member who can take my calls if you are not available?

- What will be the schedule of follow-up visits after the operation?

- What amount of time will I need to take off from work?

- How long before I can go out in public without anyone noticing I've had surgery?

- When can I bathe?

- When can I drive?

- When can I start exercising? Are there restrictions?

- When can I resume having sexual relations?

- How long should the healing take?

- How will I feel emotionally after surgery?

- What happens if I don't like the result?

- For the procedure I am considering, how often do you have to go back for a second surgery to correct/revise something?

- What is your revision policy? Who pays for that? If I need any revisions, how long after the initial surgery would I have to wait?

CHAPTER 4

Paying for Cosmetic Surgery

Cosmetic Surgery Fees

Cosmetic surgery has become remarkably affordable as the field of plastic/ cosmetic surgery has gotten more competitive and many people have decided that aesthetic enhancements are a good way to spend some of their disposable income. Also, with the use of credit cards and medical financing, a facelift could be as little as $150 per month. A number of financial components make up the cost of cosmetic surgery.

PHYSICIANS' FEES

Physicians' fees vary greatly across the country and even within a geographical area or city. Overhead expenses, the physician's experience, the geographic area, the laws of supply and demand, and what the market will bear can all be determining factors.

Potential patients need to be aware of the following:

- Just because a physician's fees are the highest does not necessarily mean that he is the best physician for your needs.

- The amount a physician charges (the most or the least) should not be a determining factor in your choice. Instead, make your choice based on whom you trust with your health, well-being, and appearance.

- If multiple procedures are being performed at the same time, some physicians have different price ranges for primary and secondary procedures.

- It is not unheard of to negotiate fees with your physician, especially if you are having multiple procedures.

- Payment in full of the surgical fees is usually required two weeks in advance or the surgery will not be performed.

- Cancellation policies usually require between 10 and 30 percent of the surgical fee to be paid if the surgery is canceled within two weeks prior to the scheduled date, unless the surgery is rescheduled. Cancellation for illness or a death in the immediate family of the patient is generally not subject to the cancellation fee if the surgery is rescheduled.

IMPLANT MATERIAL FEES

The cost of implant materials for augmentation of the breasts, calves, cheeks, chin, lips, and so on may be quoted separately or could be included in the surgical or facility fee. Make sure that you ask whether this cost is included so that you are not surprised with additional costs afterwards.

FACILITY FEES

Cosmetic surgery is performed in hospitals, outpatient facilities, and physicians' own surgical centers. Fees can vary accordingly.

- There is usually a set fee per procedure, determined by the amount of time and supplies involved. For example, a face-lift may take eight units of time, whereas upper eyelid surgery may take only six units of time. The time could also vary by doctor.

- If multiple procedures are being performed at the same time, some facilities have a primary and secondary procedure(s) price range. There generally is a price advantage to scheduling more than one procedure at one time. Using the above example, if you were to schedule both a face-lift and eyelid surgery, the facility fees might be offered at eleven or twelve units of time, instead of the combined single unit price of fourteen. The facility is already set up for surgery and can offer you savings in this manner.

- Some surgical facilities (if they are a separate entity from the physician) do not accept credit cards; some do not accept personal or business checks. Call ahead and find out what type of payment they do accept.

- If the procedure or a portion of the procedure may be reimbursed by insurance, find out if you can save money by paying cash in advance. There may be a difference in the cash versus insurance price.

- Preregister and pay for the surgical facility in advance of your surgery. Many outpatient facilities will not allow the surgery to proceed if payment has not been received in advance. Check with your facility about its policy.

ANESTHESIOLOGIST FEES

These fees are quoted as estimates and may or may not be a part of the facility charges. You may receive additional billing(s), depending on the actual length of your procedure and the supplies used. (This may not apply if your surgery is to be performed in the physician's own surgical suite.)

LAB FEES

Most physicians require certain lab tests to determine your health prior to surgery. The type and extent of the tests, e.g., blood work, chest x-ray, electrocardiogram (EKG), or eye exam, are determined by the type of surgery to be performed, your medical history, and the physician's preference. For the lab tests, you may go to your family doctor, an independent lab, or a hospital facility. Your surgeon's office may arrange for these tests.

AVERAGE SURGICAL FEES

On the next page are average ranges for cosmetic surgery procedures. These fees do *not* include the facility and anesthesia fees.

AVERAGE FACILITY FEES

Facility fees are in addition to the fees listed above. Surgical facility fees vary according to the geographic area, the type of facility, the patients' needs, and the number and type of procedures. Generally, when several procedures are performed, a price break on the facility fees is offered.

OVERNIGHT STAYS

Most cosmetic procedures can be performed on an outpatient basis. Certain procedures, e.g., abdominoplasty (tummy tuck), may require an overnight stay. Having multiple procedures or lack of home care services or coming from out of town might make an overnight stay advisable. Often, the surgical suite or outpatient facility has overnight accommodations. If not, a nearby hotel can generally serve you well. The cost in an outpatient or surgical facility complete

AVERAGE SURGICAL FEES

PROCEDURE	SURGICAL FEES
Abdominoplasty (tummy tuck)	$4,000–$5,500
Blepharoplasty (upper and lower eyelids)	$3,000–$4,030
Botox injection (per session)	$400–$500
Brachioplasty (arm lift)	$2,500–$3,000
Breast augmentation (does *not* include the cost of implants)	$1,850–$2,900
Breast lift (mastopexy)	$3,600–$4,070
Breast reduction (mammaplasty)	$6,200–$7,000
Brow/forehead lift	$2,300–$3,750
Cheek augmentation (does *not* include the cost of implants)	$1,800–$3,000
Chin augmentation (does *not* include the cost of implants)	$1,200–$1,925
Collagen injection—per cubic centimeter (cc)	$300–$350
Dermapigmentation (cosmetic tattooing or permanent make-up)	
Eyebrows	$400–$900
Eyeliner	$500–$800
Lips	$500–$800
Areola	$500–$600
Male breast reduction	$2,100–$3,000
Laser resurfacing—carbon dioxide laser (CO_2)—full face	$2,400–$3,850
Liposuction (varies according to the amount to be reduced)	
Chin-neck	$1,350–$2,000
Abdomen	$1,400–$3,000
Thighs	$1,800–$3,600
Knees	$700–$1,500
Ankles	$1,400–$2,400
Arms	$1,000–$2,600
Hips	$1,400–$2,000
Otoplasty (ear pinning)	$2,200–$3,000
Rhinoplasty (nose reshaping)	$3,200–$6,500
Rhytidectomy (face-lift)	$4,400–$6,720

Note: To learn more about fees in specific geographic regions, you may want to access the following Web sites:

American Society of Plastic and Reconstructive Surgeons at www.plasticsurgery.org

American Academy of Cosmetic Surgery at www.cosmeticsurgery.org

with private-duty nursing care can range from $400 to $600 per night. You may be able to save money if you arrange for a hotel room and pay separately for private-duty nursing care.

PRIVATE-DUTY NURSING CARE FEES

Depending upon the extent of surgery and the level of help at home, it is recommended that you hire outside assistance at least for the first night after surgery. Private-duty nursing care administered by a registered nurse (R.N.) may range from $25 to $50 per hour. A licensed practical nurse (LPN) may charge $15 to $18 per hour. At the very least, you should consider companion care at a cost of $8 to $12 per hour. If your friends offer their services, have at least two shifts for the first twenty-four hours so that each of your caregivers can get some rest and be alert to your needs.

Insurance Billing for Cosmetic Procedures

A few cosmetic surgery procedures, such as breast reconstruction, breast reduction, and hernia repair in conjunction with an abdominoplasty, may be reimbursed by your insurance company. However, most insurance companies require predetermination prior to surgery to ascertain the amount of coverage, if any. Your doctor's office may offer to submit the appropriate paperwork to your insurance company. Some doctors do not offer this service, in which case you will need to handle the paperwork associated with insurance reimbursement.

If the procedure may be reimbursed by insurance, be aware that some surgical facilities have a "cash" price and an "insurance" price. You may want to consider paying the "cash" price up front and then submit the bill to your insurance company for reimbursement. In this way, you may ultimately end up paying less for your portion of the bill. Your physician's office may be able to guide you. We have encountered facilities that actually charge two to three times more than the cash price, because of the administration involved with insurance reimbursement. This could result in additional out-of-pocket expense for you. Even if your portion is 10, 20, or 30 percent of the bill, you still want your cost to be as reasonable as possible.

Some functional procedures may be performed in conjunction with cosmetic procedures. For example, many patients have a rhinoplasty (nose reshaping) performed at the same time as a septoplasty (repair of the underlying nasal structure). The septoplasty is a functional procedure and may be insurance reimbursable. However, the rhinoplasty would not be reimbursed because it is a cosmetic procedure. Be wary if your doctor offers you the opportunity to have a cosmetic procedure along with a functional procedure and tells you that both will be billed to insurance. Move on to another doctor, since this is insurance fraud and you both could be subject to legal repercussions.

Financing Cosmetic Surgery

Years ago, finance companies never would have thought of financing face-lifts. The problem primarily was how to repossess a cosmetic surgical procedure (unlike a car) if a patient defaulted on the payments.

All of that has changed as traditional and medical finance companies have realized the size of the cosmetic surgery market. Depending on your credit history and ability to pay, many companies may be willing to help you pay for the "new you." Your payments could be as low as $150 per month, with a small down payment.

Be advised, however, that cosmetic surgery financing fees can be quite high, even compared to credit card fees. Also be aware that if you call a finance company, you will be referred to one of the company's "member" doctors. Finance companies vary in the kinds of credentials they require of their members— many do not even require board certification. So even if you find a doctor who will agree to finance your procedure, you must still check his credentials carefully. (See "Patient Financing Companies" in the Resource section on page 275.)

CHAPTER 5

Preparing for Surgery and Recovery

Smoking

As you well know, smoking is detrimental to your health. The same may be true for secondary smoke. Smoking is even more detrimental to your recovery after any type of surgical procedure.

The nicotine in cigarettes or cigars causes the blood vessels to constrict, which reduces the flow of blood. When blood flow is reduced, oxygen to the skin is decreased, and optimal healing may not take place. In extreme cases, the effect is abnormal or exaggerated scarring, or the skin can die and turn black, a condition known as skin necrosis.

The current recommendation by most surgeons is to discontinue smoking a minimum of two weeks pre- and postsurgery. There are some physicians who choose not to perform aesthetic surgeries on smokers.

If you know that you will have some difficulty quitting smoking (even for the minimum four-week period), consult with your family physician and ask for a physician-recommended smoking-cessation program.

Please do yourself a favor—QUIT!

Products Containing Aspirin and Ibuprofen

Prior to surgery (usually for a minimum of two weeks), your physician will likely advise you to discontinue the use of any products containing aspirin or ibuprofen. Use of these products can interfere with the natural clotting ability of the blood and make surgery more difficult and dangerous. The following is a partial list of some of these products. It does not include any generic preparations sold under store brands or other names. It is of utmost importance that you check with your doctor concerning any medications you take, whether prescription or over-the-counter. Your pharmacist can also assist you with information about any product of which you may be unsure.

Advil
Alka-Seltzer tablets
Alka-Seltzer Plus Cold Medicine
Anacin capsules and tablets
A.P.C. tablets
Anacin Maximum Strength
Arthritis Pain Formula (Anacin)
Arthritis Strength Bufferin
Ascriptin
Aspergum
Aspirin suppositories
Bayer Aspirin
Bayer Children's Chewable Aspirin
Bayer Children's Cold Tablets
Buff-A tablets
Bufferin
Cama Tabs
Cetased, Improved
Congespirin
Coricidin D decongestant tablets
Coricidin for children
Coricidin Demilets tablets for
    children
Coricidin tablets
Darvon
Darvon-N
Dristan decongestant
Ecotrin tablets
Empirin
Empirin with Codeine
Emprazil tablets
Emprazil-C tablets En Tab
Excedrin
Extra-Strength Bufferin

Fiorinal
Fiorinal with Codeine
Gemnisyn
Goody's Headache Powders
Medipren
Midol
Momentum Muscular Backache
    Formula
Motrin
Norgesic
Norgesic Forte
Norwich Aspirin
Nuprin
Pabirin buffered tablets
Panalgesic
Percodan and Percodan-Demi
    tablets
Quiet World Analgesic/
    Sleeping Aid
Robaxisal tablets
SK-65 Compound
Sine-Off Sinus Medicine
Stanback
Supac
Synalgos-DC capsules
Triaminicin tablets
Vanquish
Verin
Viro-Med tablets
ZORprin

Source: *Physicians Desk Reference*

Recovery Period

Everyone reacts differently to life's experiences. The same is true for those undergoing cosmetic surgery. An individual's emotional and physical health can play a large role in the recovery process. Additionally, the following critical factors can influence how a patient heals and determine the results that can be expected:

- thorough and careful preoperative evaluation
- preparation
- an experienced and skilled surgeon
- patient compliance with the doctor's instructions
- quality follow-up care

Numerous studies have shown a definite correlation between informed patients and faster recoveries. If you are mentally prepared and physically ready for a cosmetic procedure (or any surgical procedure), your recovery period can be easier and shorter. Make sure you discuss what to expect before, during, and after surgery with your doctor and/or the patient advocate if the doctor employs such a staff member. (A patient advocate assists the doctor with patient questions and other needs during the cosmetic surgery process.)

Ask to speak with other patients who have had the same procedure you are considering. If the doctor is reluctant to give names and a confidential way for you to contact former patients, you may want to consult with another doctor. Remember—most doctors are likely to refer you only to patients who have had excellent results. This is only to be expected. However, you will find that most patients will be very honest and open about their experiences. Ask them about anything that concerns you—they are lay people, just like you. They can talk to you on a personal level about any of your anxieties and apprehensions. They will likely be more than happy to share any tips they discovered as they went through the process of preparing for surgery and postoperative recuperation.

HEALING

Many things affect the length of the initial healing period:

- the type and extent of procedure(s)
- a patient's adherence to the physician's instructions

- a patient's genetics
- a patient's physical and emotional well-being
- if a patient smokes and/or drinks alcohol
- a patient's pain tolerance

Just as a machine needs to be in optimal condition to run smoothly and efficiently, so does the body. It requires a lot of energy to heal. Before and after surgery, be sure to get plenty of rest, drink lots of water, eat a healthy diet, and take medications as prescribed. This is not the time to diet, but you may consider reducing your fat and carbohydrate grams. It is also important to reduce your sodium intake as much as possible. Sodium makes the body retain fluid, causing the tissues to swell (edema). Some physicians recommend a complete elimination of sodium from the diet in the first few weeks following surgery.

PAIN

The majority of people go through the recovery period without incident. However, what one person may deem as mild discomfort, another person may perceive as pain. Tylenol may be all that is necessary to alleviate any discomfort for some; others may require prescription pain medication. Do not be afraid to take your pain medications as prescribed—your surgeon does not want you to be uncomfortable. However, be aware that pain medication can cause grogginess and a "disconnected" feeling that, for some people, may be more uncomfortable than the pain or discomfort. Some individuals have reported that they felt much better once they stopped taking the pain medication. Ultimately, you need to be the judge.

CONSTIPATION

Pain medication and inactivity slow down the normal activity of the intestinal tract and can cause constipation. It is critical not to strain during elimination, especially if you have had any procedure to the head, neck, or abdomen. If you tend to have a problem with constipation, speak with your physician prior to surgery regarding a laxative or stool softener. Eating plenty of whole grains, fresh or dried fruits and vegetables, and/or drinking prune juice may be all that is necessary for you. And don't forget to drink a lot of water (at least eight glasses per day).

DEPRESSION

Some patients experience a brief period of depression a week to a month after cosmetic surgery. This is not unusual and is only temporary. This depression may be determined by several factors, including the ones listed below:

- unrealistic expectations—not only concerning the outcome, but also the necessary preparations, the actual surgery, the recovery period, and the discomfort

- the reason(s) for having cosmetic surgery—patients who have cosmetic surgery to please someone else may be at greater risk for developing postoperative psychological complications

- the level of support and help from friends and family

- changes in normal routine

- decreased activity level

- lack of socializing and going out in public during the initial healing period

- medications used during surgery and postoperatively

- changes in self-concept

All of these factors may have a tremendous effect on the mind and body. Short-term, mild depression is perfectly normal. If it extends beyond several weeks and becomes severe, contact your surgeon's office. The doctor may refer you to a therapist or counselor. If you currently visit with a counselor, discuss your upcoming surgery and any anxieties in detail.

PLANNING FOR SURGERY

There is no such thing as preparing too much for this experience. Plan, plan, plan—do whatever it takes to minimize, if not eliminate, any anxiety, stress, or feelings of being out of control. And do not be afraid to ask for help from your friends or family. Every moment spent planning will pay off in a faster and easier recovery.

CHAPTER 6

Taking Care of Your Skin

Skin Types

The type of skin you have can determine whether you are a good candidate for cosmetic surgery. Typically, fair-skinned people are better candidates because fair skin has less of a tendency to scar. However, darker-skinned people usually age more gracefully because their skin tends to be thicker or more plump, which staves off the wrinkles longer. The basic skin type cannot be changed with creams or lotions. Skin type is a God-given characteristic that makes all of us wonderfully unique. No skin type is better than another; however, because of your skin type your doctor may work with you differently than another person. Different skin types are another reason to make sure you do not select your doctor based on the results that your friend or neighbor had. Each patient is different and may require a different approach—and even a different doctor.

WHICH ONE ARE YOU?

Skin is classified by the manner in which it is affected by sunlight.

Type I—Very fair, often freckled. People with type I skin have blond or red hair and blue or green eyes. This type of skin always burns, never tans, becomes more freckled with exposure to sun.

Type II—Pale, lightly pigmented. People with type II skin have blond to brown hair and blue, green, or brown eyes. This type of skin burns first, then tans with some freckling.

Type III—Medium-toned olive or beige skin. People with type III skin have brown to black hair and usually brown eyes. This type of skin may sometimes burn, but it tans well and rarely freckles.

Type IV—Dark olive to light brown skin. People with type IV skin have brown to black hair and brown eyes. This type of skin rarely burns, tans quickly and darkly and never freckles.

Type V—Medium to dark brown skin. People with type V skin have dark brown to black hair and brown eyes. This type of skin never burns, always tans.

Type VI—Very dark brown to black skin. People with type VI skin have black hair and dark brown or black eyes. This type of skin never burns, always tans.

DEFINITIONS OF SCARRING/SKIN CHANGES

These terms for skin changes are used throughout the book, but especially in part 2. Keep these definitions in mind or refer back to this section as you read.

Hypertrophic scarring—a raised scar, usually nodular and red.

Keloid scarring—an extreme version of hypertrophic scarring; the scar is not only elevated, but also spreading in a "clawlike" fashion.

Hyperpigmentation—darkening of the skin that may or may not be permanent.

Hypopigmentation—lightening of the skin; this condition can occur as a result of laser resurfacing, but unlikely.

ETHNIC CONSIDERATIONS

When choosing your doctor, questions should be asked about his experience with different ethnic populations, if this applies to you. Learning about your doctor's training and experience is critical because of how surgery might affect the healing of different skin types.

- Asians, African Americans, and Hispanics generally have more supple skin than Caucasians and tend to wrinkle less and age more slowly.

- Liposuction is usually very successful for Asians, African Americans, and Hispanics because their skin tends to "re-drape" well.

- Dark skin is thicker and may be prone to hyperpigmentation, keloids, and hypertrophic scarring. However, it is a myth that all Asian or African American patients develop keloids or pigmentation problems after surgery.

- If a patient has a history of hypertrophic scarring or keloids, elective cosmetic surgery should be undertaken with extreme caution or avoided. The decision to proceed must be made with a physician who is aware of the tendency to scar.

- Dark-skinned patients who do not have a history of scarring problems and show a good healing response can feel comfortable seeking cosmetic surgery.

- It is especially important to seek out a surgeon who is specially trained and/or experienced in working with ethnic populations or patients who have dark skin.

- A very careful and thorough assessment by the patient's physician is an absolute necessity.

- With laser resurfacing, chemical peels, and dermabrasion, patients with dark skin may run the risk of hyperpigmentation and scarring. They may not be a good candidate for these procedures.

- The erbium laser has been used successfully on patients with darker skins. The erbium laser penetrates less deeply than the CO_2 or other chemical/manual procedures. Check with your physician.

- Some areas of the body, such as the back and sternum, are more prone to hypertrophic scarring.

- To our knowledge, there has been no documented case of hypertrophic scarring in the mid-face area.

MALE CONSIDERATIONS

Since more and more men are undergoing cosmetic surgery, the special qualities of male skin need to be kept in mind.

- Men tend to have thicker skin than women.

- A man's facial area usually contains hair, which means the blood supply is greater. This could result in a greater risk of bleeding. However, the increased blood supply may facilitate healing.

Skin Care for Facial Procedures

Good skin care is an integral part of successful cosmetic surgery. Additionally, it ensures the long-term maintenance of the results achieved by surgery. In this chapter you will find both general and specific tips for skin care. To begin, let's review the definition of healthy skin:

- freedom from congestion (blocked pores, whiteheads, blackheads)
- a moderate to rapid cell turnover rate
- even coloration
- moderate to firm tone
- the ability to hold water efficiently

As skin ages, it naturally loses its ability to hold water, and skin cell exfoliation slows significantly. It is now known that improving both cell turnover and water retention rates will enhance postsurgical wound healing.

PRIOR TO SURGERY

The condition of your skin may be evaluated by an esthetician (licensed skin care specialist) and/or dermatologist. Upon evaluation, recommendations may be made to correct, enhance, or maintain healthy skin functions. Following these recommendations can enhance the healing process immediately after your surgery and support long-term results.

RECOVERY PERIOD

The first ten to fourteen days following your surgery is called the recovery period. During this time your doctor will give you specific directions on how to care for incision lines, laser-resurfaced skin, swelling, bruising, or other wound healing. The focus of this period is on wound healing and the avoidance of secondary infection. Therefore, you must follow your physician's specific instructions in relation to your surgical recovery. Your daily skin care during this period should focus on gentle cleansing and moisturizing.

AFTER YOUR RECOVERY PERIOD

You will begin to learn new habits pertaining to the long-term care of your skin. Along with skin care products, a change of lifestyle habits may be beneficial. For example, stopping smoking, decreasing sun exposure, limiting alcohol consumption, and getting adequate sleep will prolong the enhanced effect of your recent cosmetic surgery.

Products such as Retin-A, alpha-hydroxy acids, and some antioxidants are usually reintroduced to your everyday routine approximately three weeks following your surgery. You should begin use of these products slowly, as your skin may be sensitive at this point in your recovery. More than likely, you will be able to tolerate your normal skin care products over time.

HEALTHY SKIN CARE OBJECTIVES

Skin care products promising magical results are everywhere, many with exorbitant price tags. Wouldn't it be refreshing to understand what you should be using on your skin and why? Also, many of the products that are suggested are available at your local drugstore at a reasonable price . The following objectives of healthy skin care will help you begin a sensible approach to gaining or maintaining youthful vibrant skin.

To Increase Cell Rejuvenation Rates— Improve the Production of Collagen

Collagen is the fibrous protein present in connective tissue including skin, bone, and dental tissue. When more collagen is present, the skin is more plump and elastic. A few brand-name products to look for are: RA, Micro-RA, Affirm, AHA (glycolic acid, lactic acid), BHA, and vitamin C (L-ascorbic acid) products such as Cellex-C. Some of these products are sold over the counter; others must be obtained either through a skin care specialist or a physician. The AHA brand can be found in the form of a cream and can be purchased over the counter at your local drugstore.

To Deeply Cleanse Pores— Remove Blackheads, Whiteheads, and Unblock Pores

The manual method is called "acne surgery" and is performed in a clinical setting by a trained dermatology nurse, dermatologist, or esthetician. The procedure is much like a facial but with extensive extractions and deeper cleaning performed. The chemical interventions include glycolic acid peels or products such as Retin-A, micro-RA, or Affirm.

To Improve Water Retention Rates

Glycolic acid has been found to be very beneficial, as it retrains the skin to hold water. Use moisturizers that contain humectants (ingredients that attract water to the skin). Be sure you are using appropriate application methods (amount of product and frequency). Glycolic acid is obtainable over the counter.

To Decrease Pigmentation Production— Balance Uneven Skin Coloration

Hydroquinone is a substance that balances skin tone and can be found in drugstore products at 2 percent strength and by prescription from 3 percent to 8 percent strength. Some physicians have their own formulas, which may be blended with Retin-A and hydrocortisone. *Note:* Because of the hydrocortisone, patients using this product are generally under the strict supervision of the physician. A series of glycolic acid peels (six to eight peels) may help control hyperpigmentation. Glycolic acid peels should only be applied by a physician or trained skin care specialist.

To Protect Skin from Sunlight

Follow these rules to be "sun smart":

- Avoid the sun between 10 A.M. and 4 P.M.

- Wear sunblock with a sun protection factor (SPF) of fifteen to fifty and re-apply it every ninety minutes when you are exposed to sun, perspiration, or water.

- Use at least two bottles of sunblock per year.

- If you are sensitive to sunblock, try a physical sunblock—sun-protective clothing such as large-brimmed hats.

The protective value of any sun protective product above SPF 30 is still in question. However, any product labeled above SPF 30 will give you at least the protective value of SPF 20 to 30, if not more. Do not pay more for higher SPF claims. Some sunscreens have hydroquinones in them. These work best if you are darker pigmented or have a tendency to tan easily.

LONG-TERM SKIN CARE GUIDELINES

Having healthy skin goes hand in hand with having a healthy body. Therefore, it is important to incorporate daily healthy skin care habits at home. You may wish to continue working under the guidance of a professional (esthetician or dermatologist) who specializes in the care of the skin.

CHAPTER 7

Patient Tips and Secrets

Numerous studies show a definite correlation between informed patients and faster recoveries. Sometimes it is the little details that can make a huge difference. This is definitely the case when it comes to cosmetic surgery. Since having cosmetic surgery is generally a once or twice-in-a-lifetime event, you wouldn't necessarily be aware of the kinds of tips and little secrets that can make your experience a positive one. The following is a collection of pointers that have been compiled from many different perspectives, as well as patients' experiences. Be sure to check with your doctor concerning any of the following tips that pertain to healing and/or medications to make sure that they are appropriate for you.

Prior to Surgery

Some preplanning can go a long way to make your recovery comfortable. It is easy to think that the time you'll be taking off is an opportunity to catch up on personal business. That may be so for some people, but don't put off some essential preparations that you could take care of prior to your surgery. Taking the time to plan can make your life easier before and after surgery. This chapter has many ideas to help you plan wisely. The tips in this section are designed to be followed approximately two to three weeks before your surgery date.

PHYSICIAN'S INSTRUCTIONS

If you cannot comply with your doctor's basic pre- and postoperative instructions, reconsider your decision to have surgery.

MEDICAL HISTORY

It is of the utmost importance that you are totally honest with your doctor regarding your medical history (including any medications you are currently taking), no matter how insignificant you may feel something is. Do not be embarrassed—your health and well-being are at stake.

COLD SORES/HERPES VIRUS

If you will be undergoing any type of facial peel, dermabrasion, or laser resurfacing, it is critical that you tell your doctor if you have a history of cold sores, shingles, or herpes infections. Most doctors routinely prescribe an oral antiviral medication. You can run the risk of severe scarring if you have a breakout after these procedures. Also indicate if you are currently taking any acne medication or have any connective tissue disease. It is also important that you supply your physician with information about previous skin peels (glycolic, lactic acid, or trichloroacetic acid/TCA) and previous facial waxing (hot or cold). Be sure to mention what type you had and when. Also discuss the skin products you are currently using (Retin-A, glycolic acids, topical vitamin C).

YEAST INFECTIONS

Generally, you are given antibiotics to stave off any infections as a result of surgery. If you are prone to yeast infections, you may want to take full-spectrum acidophilus ("good bacteria") supplements. They can be found in any health food store.

SMOKING

If you smoke, you MUST quit a minimum of two weeks pre- and postoperatively. Some surgeons will not perform surgery on a smoker who has not committed to the minimum quitting period because of concerns about scarring and healing complications.

ALCOHOL

Discontinue alcohol consumption a minimum of two weeks pre- and postoperatively. It is imperative that you are totally honest with your physician and anesthesiologist if you have consumed any alcohol within this time period, so that your anesthesia medications can be adjusted.

NUTRITION

If you don't already eat in a healthy way, it would be a very good idea to start now. This will help ensure proper healing and tissue repair.

MENSTRUATION

Consider speaking with your doctor about scheduling your surgery with regard to your menstrual period. If you routinely take ibuprofen to control cramps, you may be asked to take a nonaspirin/nonibuprofen analgesic instead. Depending on the severity of your menstrual cramping, scheduling of surgery accordingly could greatly increase your comfort during recovery.

SURGICAL FACILITY FEES—PAYMENT AND INSURANCE

Some surgical facilities (separate from the physician) do not accept credit cards; some do not accept personal or business checks. Call ahead and find out what type of payment they do accept before you go to prepay.

PREREGISTRATION AT THE SURGICAL FACILITY

Preregister and pay for the surgical facility in advance of your surgery. Do not wait until the day of your surgery—you will have enough to think about. Also, many outpatient facilities will not allow the surgery to proceed if payment has not been received in advance.

FEE ESTIMATES VERSUS ACTUAL FEES

Remember, the facility and anesthesiologist fees you pay prior to surgery are estimates. You may receive additional billing(s), depending on the actual length of your procedure and the supplies used. (This may not apply if your surgery is to be performed in the physician's own surgical suite).

HERBAL SUGGESTIONS

Many doctors today are recommending *Arnica montana*. It is considered a safe and natural homeopathic remedy and can be purchased at most herb shops. If you take it once a day for two weeks before and after surgery, you may experience much less bruising than you would normally, and the bruising may diminish more rapidly. It is available in a pill and cream form. Contact your physician or speak to a professional in the herbal/homeopathic field.

HAIR CARE PRIOR TO SURGERY (COLOR OR PERMANENTS)

If you wish to color your hair or have a permanent, do so a minimum of ten days to three weeks prior to surgery if your procedure involves sutures in your scalp area. It will be four to six weeks after surgery before you can color your hair or have a permanent again. This may also apply to laser resurfacing or chemical peels. Check with your doctor.

HOUSEKEEPING PRIOR TO SURGERY

Prior to surgery, pay your bills, clean your house thoroughly, care for your plants and yard, change the sheets on your bed and generally make sure your life is in order. You won't feel like doing housework for at least a week and possibly two (depending on the procedures) after the surgery.

AVOIDANCE OF SODIUM AND OTHER SUBSTANCES

When you go to the grocery store prior to your surgery, read product labels and avoid spicy foods and products high in sodium. A no-salt diet is usually recommended to prevent swelling/fluid retention (edema) for at least a week to ten days prior to surgery. Also avoid caffeine and alcohol according to your doctor's recommendations.

MEAL PREPARATION

You may want to prepare some meals ahead of time and freeze them. For at least the first few days after surgery, you will not feel like cooking. If you have had facial procedures, make sure the food is easy to chew and not too crunchy. You need to avoid excess facial movements for the first few days of your recovery.

HEAD ELEVATION

If your physician has instructed that your head and upper body need to be elevated, put pillowcases on at least four extra pillows—two to prop up your head and one to place on each side of you so that you can't turn on your side while sleeping. If you have had a body procedure or have lower back problems, you may want an extra pillow to put under or between your knees.

PAIN MEDICATION

Fill all of your prescriptions in advance. You may not need your pain medication, but if you do, you won't want to have to wait while someone goes to get it.

ASPIRIN/IBUPROFEN PRODUCTS

Discontinue aspirin or any products containing aspirin or ibuprofen (see list on page 50) at least two weeks prior to surgery and two weeks after surgery. Aspirin interferes with your body's blood-clotting mechanism.

VITAMIN USAGE

Discontinue taking vitamin E a minimum of two weeks prior to surgery and for two weeks after surgery. Starting two weeks prior to surgery and continuing through the two weeks after surgery, consider taking a multivitamin supplement and a minimum of 500 milligrams of vitamin C twice daily. Ask your doctor what products would be best for you.

COMPRESSION GARMENTS AFTER LIPOSUCTION

If you are having body liposuction or an abdominoplasty, most doctors require that you wear a compression garment for four to six weeks. Excellent sources are Macy's, Kmart, and JCPenney. An alternative is lycra bicycle shorts.

Preparing for Surgery

ANESTHESIA

Be sure to tell the doctor and the anesthesiologist if you are prone to nausea, allergic to any medications, or if you or any of your immediate family members have ever had any kind of reaction to anesthesia.

NIGHT-LIGHT

Get a night-light for when you get up in the middle of the night, so you won't trip or fall.

CHILDCARE

Young children will not understand that they cannot jump in your lap or be lifted up after surgery. Make sure that you have some assistance and do your best to explain that you must be careful for the first part of your recovery.

PET INTERACTION AND CARE

You may consider your pets a part of your family; however, you do need to keep them from licking you on or near your incisions. Do not lift your pets or bend over to feed them. After petting your pet, wash your hands with soap and water before touching your surgical area(s). Try to keep your pets off your bedding and anywhere you will be sitting while recuperating to avoid opportunistic germs.

CAREGIVER COMFORT AND INSTRUCTIONS

Borrow a baby monitor for the first forty-eight hours. In that way, whoever is staying with you does not have to stay in the same room with you the entire time. Write down all instructions, including what medications you are supposed to take and when. This is for your caregiver and also you (so you don't forget). Place your doctor's name and telephone number, along with your pharmacy information, in a conspicuous place.

SUPPLIES

In advance, lay out all medications and any supplies needed, such as Q-Tips, hydrogen peroxide, and gauze pads, in an easily accessible place.

DRESSINGS FOR FACE-LIFT, BROW LIFT, FACIAL IMPLANTS, OTOPLASTY

For some facial procedures, a "mummy wrap" will probably be applied. Depending on the procedure, your entire head may be covered with a dressing, perhaps as large as a football helmet (a number of variations of dressings are utilized). It must remain in place until the physician or nurse removes it (one day to a few days). If you become claustrophobic, inform your doctor so that he can keep the dressing as loose as possible where it passes under your chin. If your skin is sensitive, ask your doctor to place a piece of soft cloth between the skin under your chin and the dressing to prevent chafing.

COLD COMPRESSES

If your doctor indicates that you are to use cold compresses, consider buying four to six packages of frozen peas and put each bag in a plastic bag, so that they won't accidentally burst open. Rotate them so that they do not lose their chill. In that way, there will always be a compress ready for use. Some doctors recommend chipped ice in a rubber glove.

BOOKS ON TAPE

Borrow or buy a portable tape player with earphones so that you can listen to audio books while you are recuperating. Libraries have a great selection, you can keep them for two weeks, and they're free. This is especially helpful if you are having eyelid surgery (your eyes may feel strained or you may have been instructed by your physician to avoid reading or watching television for the first few days).

SUNGLASSES AND CONTACT LENSES

If you are having eyelid surgery, make sure you have sunglasses and/or clip-on sunglasses for your regular glasses because your eyes may be light-sensitive and feel strained. Oversized dark goggles that fit right over your glasses are available in many stores. Some doctors recommend not wearing glasses directly after a rhinoplasty (nose reshaping). Follow your doctor's advice.

If you are having eyelid surgery, your doctor will advise you not to wear contact lenses for approximately five to ten days. Follow your doctor's instructions.

VIDEOS/MAGAZINES/LETTER WRITING

You may want to catch up on all those videos you've been wanting to see (once your eyes are not bothering you if you have had eyelid surgery), magazines that have stacked up unread, letters, or the great novel you've been meaning to write. Perhaps your friends would like a letter from you about your terrific surgical experience!

BRUISING AND SWELLING

If you are having any kind of facial surgery, prepare your spouse, significant other, children, friends, and/or caregivers with the knowledge that your face will initially be swollen and bruised. Otherwise, this can be quite a shock for some people.

DRAINAGE AFTER LIPOSUCTION

If you are going to have liposuction, you may want to prepare your bed with a plastic liner (a garbage bag split up the middle will do) and an old towel. There will be drainage (the tumescent anesthesia solution) from your incisions for approximately the first twenty-four hours, and it may seep through your compression garment.

BREAST SURGERY—UNDERGARMENT COMFORT

If you are having any type of breast surgery, purchase front-closure bras to wear after your surgical bra or dressing is removed. This will minimize motion when you are dressing and undressing.

MAMMOGRAM BEFORE AND AFTER BREAST SURGERY

For any type of breast surgery, anyone who has regular mammograms or is over the age of forty should schedule a mammogram prior to the procedure and then again after the swelling and tenderness have disappeared completely (three to six months). In this way, the changes from your surgery will be documented.

TYLENOL PM/EXCEDRIN P.M.

You may want to have some Tylenol PM or Excedrin P.M. on hand for two reasons. After surgery, instead of sleeping pills, this medication may provide a restful sleep without putting you into a deep, drugged sleep. Also, these products contain a substance similar to Benadryl, which can help alleviate any itching as you heal. They can be taken every three to four hours.

The Day of Surgery

The big day is here. Often surgery takes place early in the morning, leaving you little time to prepare if you haven't done so already. At this point, stress and anxiety are normal, but you don't want to add to it by being disorganized. Ease and comfort are what you are looking for, from your clothes to your hair and personal belongings. For your hair care on the day of surgery, if you are required to wash your hair with PHisoDerm prior to surgery, deep condition your hair before you wash it. You'll also want to wear comfortable, oversized clothing, a top that buttons down the front, no bra, no makeup, and no jewelry. The nurses will probably be helping you get dressed after surgery and (trust us) you will not care what you look like after surgery. Also, travel light. Don't bother bringing your purse with you—you don't need it. Place your identification in a pocket that closes with a button or Velcro in clothing that you will be wearing home.

After Surgery

After surgery is when your perception of your cosmetic surgery experience really begins. This is the time when all of your research and planning will pay off. Your initial state or feeling upon coming out of anesthesia will depend on the type administered and your normal reaction or tolerance to it. If you've experienced anesthesia prior to your cosmetic surgery, you may recall how you felt upon waking. Although the feeling varies for everyone, most report some level of grogginess and discomfort. Because of this, the following tips will make your ride home or overnight stay easier to handle.

THE DRIVE HOME

The vehicle you will be driven home in needs to be comfortable and have good air conditioning/heat, depending on the season. If the vehicle is a four-door model, sit in the back seat. If an accident occurs, you would not want to be in the way of an air bag if it deploys—but do wear the lap and shoulder belts. If the vehicle does not have four doors, sit in the front and keep a pillow in front of you. Make sure that whoever is going to drive you home after surgery is responsible, mature, and a good driver. You do not want to be jostled around.

FOLLOW INSTRUCTIONS

Follow your doctor's instructions to the letter. If the instructions are not clear or you don't understand something—*ask*.

PAMPER YOURSELF

The postoperative period is a time to pamper yourself and rest so that you can heal (your preparations need to facilitate that). However, remember you are not sick. Follow your doctor's instructions, of course, but you will feel better the sooner you can return to a normal (though not strenuous) routine. Consider treating yourself to an in-home massage, pedicure, or foot massage.

RELIEF FOR YOUR CAREGIVER

If your doctor instructs you to apply cold compresses, be aware that (depending on the procedure) they should be applied for twenty minutes every hour for the first forty-eight hours after surgery. In other words, your caregiver will have to be up all night. Consider having two to three caregivers so that they can take shifts. Also consider having private-duty nursing care.

OVERNIGHT STAY

If possible, and if you can afford it, stay over the first night at the surgical facility or hire someone to stay with you.

FIRST NIGHT AFTER SURGERY

Even if you cannot afford to hire a caregiver, you must have, and need, someone to stay with you through the first night after surgery.

SLEEP/REST

After surgery, expect to sleep the first day. On the second day, most doctors require a postoperative visit, and that is all you should or will want to do that day. For the third and fourth days, you can expect to feel more energetic. However, you still need to rest as much as possible in a reclining position.

CALLS TO THE DOCTOR

Report anything unusual to the doctor's office immediately, i.e., nausea, vomiting, bleeding, unusual swelling (other than what you have been told to expect).

FLUID CONSUMPTION

Drink plenty of fluids, especially water. According your physician's instructions, do not consume alcohol or caffeine. For at least the first week of recuperation, have a glass of water with a bendable straw on your bedside table at all times, especially at night. Do not use a straw for about a week if you have had a facelift. Cold ginger ale is very soothing if you are nauseated from the anesthesia or if your throat hurts.

FACIAL MOVEMENT AND EATING AFTER A FACE-LIFT

If you have had a face-lift, talk through your teeth and avoid laughing, heavy chewing, and turning your head for about one week. If you must turn your head, rotate your entire torso along with your head. If you need (or want) to talk on the telephone, you may want to consider using a speakerphone. After any cosmetic surgery, your diet should be soft, bland, and light (frozen drinks are great). Remember, salty and spicy foods cause fluid retention. With most facial surgery, it's a good idea to stay on a soft diet for seventy-two hours.

BENDING OVER/STRAINING

If you have had any type of surgery to the head or neck, do not bend over. If you need to pick up anything from the floor, squat, keeping your head level. Do not pick up anything heavier than a small telephone book. Do not do anything that will raise your blood pressure.

HEAD ELEVATION

With head or facial surgery, you will need to sleep propped up and on your back. If you want to turn just the lower part of your body (hips and legs), you may be more comfortable if you place a pillow between your knees.

PILLOW PLACEMENT

If you have had liposuction on your knees and you are lying on your side, place a pillow between your knees (they can be sensitive because they are "bonier" than the rest of your leg).

COTTON GLOVES

If you are prone to scratching yourself while sleeping, purchase cotton gloves to wear at night.

ASSISTANCE WITH LIPOSUCTION GARMENTS

If your doctor has instructed you to wear a body garment, it will be much easier to put on if you shake talcum powder or cornstarch inside it. Do not be alone in the house the first time you take your liposuction garment off—you may be shaky or weak-kneed. Minimally, have someone in the next room.

BATHS

Baths can be soothing, both for your body and your psyche. However, ask your physician if and when they are permitted.

INCISIONS/SURGICAL AREAS

Use caution and a gentle touch in and around any surgical/incision areas. Do not apply anything to these areas unless you have been specifically instructed to do so by your physician.

HAIR CARE TECHNIQUES AFTER FACIAL SURGERY

Follow safe hair-washing techniques once your physician has given you permission to wash your hair after facial/neck procedures.

- Rinse hair with medium-temperature water for about five minutes prior to washing your hair. This will soften any remaining dried blood, as well as rinse out any saline that may have been used to rinse your hair immediately after surgery. Shampoo delicately with a gentle fragrance- and color-free shampoo, such as Johnson's Baby Shampoo, Tri E-Collagen Shampoo, or DHS Clear (Person & Covey). Rinse well. Stand under the shower and allow the water to gently rinse your hair. Avoid rubbing suture lines. Stay in the shower longer than usual, if necessary. Make sure the water temperature is not too hot.

- Apply conditioner (color- and fragrance-free) mainly on hair ends for detangling purposes. Examples include DHS Conditioner (Person & Covey), Paul Mitchell—The Conditioner. Do *not* apply on or near staples/sutures. Since you will be avoiding sensitive areas when you apply conditioner, you can be more flexible about product selection.

- Gently towel dry hair as much as possible. Then clean both staple and suture lines with hydrogen peroxide (or as directed by your physician).

- You won't feel much like styling your hair as you normally do. Plan to wear scarves or gently tie or clip your hair back for the first few days. Avoid excessive tension—tight headbands, pulling hair back severely, clips too close to the suture/staple lines, and so on. These styling methods may compromise wound healing. *Be careful!*

- Do not wash your hair for twenty-four hours *after* staples have been removed. This time will allow your skin to heal. You *may* wash your hair *prior* to your appointment(s) for staple removal.

- Your hair may feel drier than usual after surgery. The use of PHisoDerm (which may have been recommended for shampooing prior to surgery by your physician) and the anesthesia contribute to drying out your hair. A deep conditioner (ten to thirty minutes) is a good idea on about day twelve. Your stylist can condition your hair, or you can do it at home. An example of a deep conditioner is Clairol 10-Minute Conditioner.

- Avoid excessive heat on and around the healing areas (hot water from the shower, blow-dryers, curling irons, curlers). Blow-dryers must be held at least twelve inches from the hair to avoid heating staples.

- Avoid excessive brushing or combing. *Be gentle.*

- Avoid any products with color or fragrance for at least two weeks following surgery (including hair spray).

FACE-WASHING TECHNIQUES

After any facial procedure, you may cleanse your face as usual. However, you must avoid scrubbing or buffing your face. Gentle cleansers such as Aquanil, Cetaphil, or CAM lotion may be used without a problem. Moisturize the surrounding skin as usual, avoiding the incision lines. Do not use astringents or toners on healing areas. Avoid AHA, Retin-A or other exfoliant-type creams on suture areas. Some physicians may suggest Retin-A to help limit any possibility of scarring. However, your physician will let you know if this is appropriate for you.

PAIN/SLEEPING MEDICATIONS

The sooner you can stop taking the pain and/or sleeping medication, the better you will feel. However, take it if necessary—your physician does not want you to be in pain.

ENERGY FOR HEALING

If you feel tired, rest—it takes a lot of energy for your body to heal.

DO NOT DIET

While recuperating, *do not diet.* Your body needs all the nutrition you can give it to have the energy to heal faster. So eat healthy foods: lots of *fresh* fruits and *fresh* vegetables (puréed if necessary), whole grains, and protein (increase your normal intake).

BEAUTY SALONS AFTER SURGERY

If you visit the beauty salon within six weeks of your surgery, avoid the hood type of hair dryer after any procedure to the face/head, including and especially laser resurfacing. Point out the location of your incisions/scars to your beauty operator. Tell him/her to be very careful with hand-held dryers and curling irons and to keep the setting on warm, not hot.

These tips and secrets have been provided to make your planning and recovery as comfortable as possible. Many of these tips come from direct patient experience and others from physicians and their staffs. Use of these pointers will vary depending upon your personal situation, but do take time to read over them at the various stages of your cosmetic surgery decision. One tip could make a difference.

Part 2

The Procedures

The detailed descriptions of the cosmetic surgery procedures presented in part 2 are designed to assist you in understanding each process and learning about your options.

You may find some of the instructions repetitious due to the similar nature of recovery for the various procedures. However, you should carefully read all of the sections for the procedures you are interested in because they contain important information that is critical to your knowledge of recovery, pre- and postoperative instructions, anesthesia, and more.

Refer back often to the sections that address the stage you are experiencing in your own cosmetic surgery process. Explore the possibilities and enjoy your learning!

*A*rm Lift–Brachioplasty

Brachioplasty is performed to eliminate excess skin from the upper arm. The procedure is also known as "arm tightening." As we age or lose a significant amount of weight, the skin of the upper arms can lose its elasticity and hang down, creating a "bat-wing deformity." With any surgical procedure, it is important to be informed. However, because of the significant scar that brachioplasty produces, it is even more important for you to educate yourself. Here are some important facts about brachioplasty.

- The procedure can be performed in conjunction with liposuction of the upper arm.

- Liposuction will reduce the amount of fat but will not eliminate the excess skin.

- Brachioplasty does produce a permanent and noticeable scar.

- The procedure is not recommended for patients with repeated underarm infections or who sweat excessively (axillary hydradenitis).

- The procedure is not recommended for mastectomy patients. It could lead to persistent swelling because the lymphatic drainage of the arm has been altered.

Procedure

Brachioplasty is not a procedure that is performed frequently because of the noticeable scar that it produces. However, if the skin has lost its elasticity, liposuction of the upper arms will not be sufficient; loose skin will remain. Some patients are willing to trade a firm upper arm for a scar. As with any procedure, ask to see the physician's before-and-after photographs of his brachioplasty patients. Remember that different doctors use different techniques and usually recommend the one(s) in which they are trained and experienced. You and your physician must take into consideration your lifestyle, the types of clothes you wear, and your desired look. In general, if you do make the decision to undergo a brachioplasty, here's what you can expect.

ANESTHESIA

A brachioplasty can be performed under local anesthesia with intravenous sedation or under general anesthesia. However, the type of anesthesia used is dependent on the procedure to be performed, the doctor's choice, and the patient's medical history or desires.

INCISIONS

Your doctor will generally mark the area of excess skin while you are standing or sitting. The incision is usually placed on the inner surface of the upper arm. It may extend from the elbow to the armpit and may be an ellipse or a triangle with the base in the axilla (armpit). Excess skin and fatty tissue are removed. However, some fat will be left to cover and protect arteries and nerves. At this time, liposuction may also be performed to achieve a smoother result. The incision is then sutured (sutures may or may not be dissolvable). A drain may be used.

STEPS IN THE ARM LIFT PROCEDURE

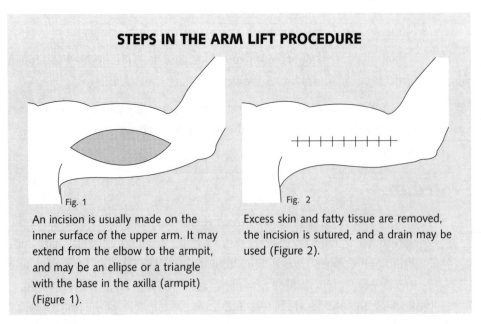

Fig. 1

An incision is usually made on the inner surface of the upper arm. It may extend from the elbow to the armpit, and may be an ellipse or a triangle with the base in the axilla (armpit) (Figure 1).

Fig. 2

Excess skin and fatty tissue are removed, the incision is sutured, and a drain may be used (Figure 2).

COMPRESSION GARMENTS/DRESSING

While you are still in the operating room, a compression garment, an absorbent bandage, or a simple dressing may be applied.

LENGTH OF PROCEDURE

A brachioplasty should take approximately two hours.

Prior to Surgery

Before surgery, you and your doctor will first make several important decisions. Then you will prepare for surgery and be given prescriptions and instructions. The following sections will give you an overview of the process.

ASSESSMENT

Your physician should evaluate and assess the location of the fat in the upper arm, along with the laxity of the skin. If there is good skin tone (elasticity), your doctor may recommend liposuction. However, if the sagging skin has lost its elasticity, brachioplasty may be recommended. Liposuction may be performed in conjunction with brachioplasty to contour the area. Be absolutely clear and in agreement with your doctor about your desired look.

LOCATION OF INCISIONS

Discuss with your physician the location of the incisions. Brachioplasty does produce a permanent and noticeable scar.

PREOPERATIVE VISIT

You should be instructed to have certain lab tests, i.e., blood work, chest x-ray, EKG. You may go to your family doctor, an independent lab, or hospital facility. The physician who will perform your surgery may arrange for the performance of these tests.

You may sign all of your surgical consent forms and be given pre- and postoperative instructions at this time. You should also be given your prescriptions for before and after surgery. Make sure that everything you and your physician have agreed to is stated on the consent form.

PRESCRIPTIONS

Some or all of these may be prescribed, in addition to others not listed.

- multivitamins—to be taken ten days to two weeks before and after surgery
- vitamin C—500 milligrams twice daily, to be taken ten days to two weeks before and after surgery
- pain medication
- antinausea medication
- oral antibiotics and/or ointment
- sleeping medication
- steroids (i.e., cortisone), to minimize swelling

Be sure to follow your doctor's instructions.

PRE- AND POSTOPERATIVE INSTRUCTIONS

These suggestions are intended to make you more comfortable and help you heal. To learn more, turn to the section on recovery in this chapter. Your doctor may have different or additional instructions. Follow them to the letter.

Stop smoking, discontinue the use of alcohol, and stop taking vitamin E and any medications containing aspirin or ibuprofen (two weeks pre- and postoperative is usually recommended). Check with your doctor regarding any other medications (including homeopathic/herbal products) that you are currently taking.

- Know how and when to take/apply your prescriptions.
- Know how to cleanse the surgical areas the night before or morning of your surgery.
- Do not have food (including gum or mints) or drink (including water) for a minimum of six to eight hours prior to surgery. (Follow your surgical facility's preoperative instructions.)
- Have someone drive you to and from surgery.
- Have someone stay with you the first night after surgery (twenty-four hours, optimally).
- If dressings and/or drains are required, they may be applied by the doctor or nurse immediately after the procedure.

- If your physician requires a compression garment, you should be instructed as to the amount of time it is to be worn (usually until the bruising and swelling have subsided). Purchase a second garment so that you always have a clean one.

- Know the directions regarding any ointments to be applied and/or cleansing of incisions.

- Do not sunbathe or use tanning beds at least two weeks prior to surgery. (For optimal skin care and health, these activities should be avoided completely.) After surgery, if you must be in the sun, protect your arms.

- Avoid aerobic activity for at least four to six weeks after surgery.

- Most physicians recommend that you get up and start taking short walks around the house by the second day, increasing the amount you walk each day.

- Avoid vigorous exercise that affects the arms for approximately six weeks.

- Do not drive for one to two weeks and while taking pain medication.

- For the first week to ten days, when lying down, lie on your back; keep your upper body and arms elevated. Place pillows to prop up your upper body and support your arms. A recliner works perfectly.

- Lift nothing heavier than a small telephone book.

- Expect some level of numbness in the areas treated for eight to twelve weeks.

- Your doctor may instruct you to apply cold compresses, usually twenty minutes every hour for a minimum of forty-eight hours.

- Rest and relax for the first week.

- As your incisions start to heal, they may itch. Do not scratch them. Ask your doctor if you can apply cream or ointment to relieve the itching and only use what is recommended.

Recovery

Everyone heals differently. Your genetics, your physical and emotional well-being, whether you smoke and/or drink alcohol, your pain tolerance, the extent of the surgery, and how well you follow the doctor's instructions affect healing. Plan on approximately one to two weeks for the initial healing period.

POSTOPERATIVE PHYSICIAN APPOINTMENTS

Your doctor may want to see you the day after surgery (if drains were inserted, they may be removed that day). That activity alone may be all you will want, or should do, that day. After your appointment, go home and rest. You may be given permission to shower that day or the next. Your sutures should be removed (if not dissolvable) around the fifth to seventh day. You should have an appointment to return to the doctor's office about three weeks after surgery and then again in six weeks, three months, and six months.

FIRST DAY POSTOPERATIVE

You may want to sleep the first day after surgery. The upper arm area may feel sore and very tight, and you may experience swelling and bruising. You will need help getting in and out of bed for the first few days. Expect some numbness and a tight feeling in the treated areas for an average of eight to twelve weeks. This feeling, however, can last up to a year.

SWELLING AND BRUISING

The bruising may last, on the average, anywhere from five days to several weeks but should diminish daily. Some minor swelling could remain after the first few weeks. If there is increased swelling and/or bruising and tenderness, this may represent a hematoma (collection of blood) under the skin. Contact your physician immediately for evaluation.

NUMBNESS AND ITCHING

You may also have some temporary numbness, which should dissipate in a maximum of six months. Also, if the incision sites itch, gently rub the areas—do not scratch them. Ask your doctor if you can apply some cream or ointment to relieve the itching and use only what is recommended.

COMPRESSION GARMENT/DRESSING

The physician or nurse may have placed compression garments on your upper arms while you were still in the operating room. They help reduce fluid buildup and support and mold the skin. Most physicians require that these garments be worn twenty-four hours a day for several weeks (usually until the bruising and swelling have subsided). They should only be removed when you shower.

COLD COMPRESSES

Cold compresses applied to the upper arm area may relieve some of the discomfort and can greatly reduce the swelling. These should be applied every hour for twenty minutes for a minimum of forty-eight hours (some doctors recommend seventy-two hours) after surgery. Ice should never be placed directly on the skin. Either use cold compresses or place a cloth between the ice bag and your skin. In some cases, your doctor may instruct you *not* to use cold compresses. Follow your doctor's instructions.

BODY POSITION

It is important that you keep your upper body propped up and your arms elevated at all times when lying down for at least the first week. Sleep on a recliner or prop yourself up with pillows. If you need to pick something up, squat with your knees bent, and do not pick up anything heavier than a small telephone book.

WALKING/EXERCISE

By the second day, you may be allowed to start taking short walks inside your house. Do not overdo it—listen to your body. If you feel tired, rest. After the first week, you may possibly resume some of your normal routine, except for strenuous activity or heavy lifting. Most physicians recommend that you wait a minimum of three to four weeks to resume aerobic exercise and six weeks for any type of upper-arm exercises.

INCISION LINES

You should receive instructions on the care of your incisions and when you can bathe. Your scars may remain red for four to six weeks. They may be wider than most scars because there is a lot of tension on the incision site due to its location. However, if the scars become raised or thickened as well as red, then notify your physician immediately. This may represent hypertrophic scarring, which can be treated.

Pain

As with recovery times, pain tolerance is different for everyone. What one person may consider pain, another person may consider discomfort.

LEVEL OF PAIN/DISCOMFORT

Generally, with brachioplasty there is minimal to moderate discomfort during the postoperative period. This usually subsides in a few days.

PAIN MEDICATION

Most discomfort can be controlled with pain medications you have been prescribed or Extra Strength Tylenol. You may find it necessary to take pain medication for the first day or two only.

Risks/Complications

Although problems are unlikely, you need to be aware of what can happen and what action you should take. Most risks/complications will be avoided if you make an informed decision, choose a qualified physician, and follow your physician's instructions.

INFECTION

If there is any serious pain, heavy oozing, or fever, these should be reported immediately to the doctor. An infection can be treated with antibiotic ointments and/or oral antibiotics.

HEMATOMA

A hematoma, a collection of blood or fluid beneath the skin, is unlikely. However, if it does occur, it can be treated by drainage with a needle or by compression.

HYPERTROPHIC SCARRING

Report any signs immediately to your doctor; this scarring can be treated if caught early. (See "Definitions of Scarring/Skin Changes" on page 56.)

SEROMA

When large amounts of fat are removed, a collection of fluid can accumulate in the space between the skin flap and muscle. If there is a leakage of clear yellow or blood-tinged fluid from the incision site, call your physician as soon as possible. The fluid can be withdrawn with a syringe. This may occur more than once.

*B*otox Injections

Botox is the trademark for the botulinum toxin A used in the injections to treat the creases on the forehead (especially between the eyebrows) and the "squinting" lines around the eyes.

It seems that every publication one picks up lately has an article concerning Botox—it's the newest rage. The average person thinks, "Everyone is doing it. How can it hurt?" However, there are consequences if Botox is not administered by an experienced physician. These consequences are not permanent, but you would have to live with them for a number of months. As with any procedure, it is extremely important for you to be totally informed. Here are some important facts about Botox.

- This procedure was used in the early 1980s to treat muscle twitching around the eyes.

- Botox is usually used on the upper third of the face.

- Botox can be injected into the corrugator and procerus muscles between the brows to treat "scowl" lines.

- Botox may also be injected to treat the "squint" lines around the eyes.

- The botulinum toxin temporarily paralyzes the muscles across the forehead and around the eyes.

- The effects can be seen within two to four days and can last from three to six months, at which time the injections can be repeated.

- Some patients experience a permanent decrease of deep lines and furrows after repeated injections.

- There is minimal discomfort during the injection. Some patients may experience a headache for three or four hours after the injection.

- This procedure can be a preliminary step to a forehead/brow lift, in which the corrugator muscles are sometimes cut to eliminate the "scowl" lines.

- Some physicians have started administering injections into the platysmal bands (muscles that go from underneath the chin to the breastbone) in the neck. These muscles may relax as one ages and have the appearance of cording.

Botox injections are in-office procedures and require no recovery time. However, improper placement of the injections can cause a temporarily "droopy" eyelid or other muscle laxity. This complication can occur if the physician is inexperienced and places the injection in the wrong muscle or if you do not follow your physician's instructions not to rub the area that received the injection. To avoid these complications, ask your physician how many times he has injected Botox and be sure to follow his instructions carefully.

*B*reast Augmentation

B reast augmentation is performed to increase the size of the breasts or to correct a difference in size between the breasts. Implants are also used to reconstruct the breast after breast cancer.

Certainly it is important to be informed about any surgical procedure. However, because we are bombarded every day with constant media attention and court cases regarding breast augmentation, it is even more important for you to be totally informed. The media always highlights the tragedies, never mentioning the millions of women who are very happy that they made the decision to have breast implants. The following section will help you sort through the often contradictory information that has been presented to the public. First, here are some interesting facts about breast augmentation.

- Breast augmentation can be performed on girls as young as their late teens, once their breasts have stopped developing.

- Breast augmentation can be performed in conjunction with a breast lift and/or reduction. The implant is placed either under or over the pectoral (chest) muscle.

- Saline implants are the main breast implant available in the United States, unless you choose to participate in a silicone gel implant clinical study. (You must go to a physician who is approved to place silicone implants.)

- No known illnesses are associated with saline-filled implants; if the saline implant ruptures, the body will absorb the saline, which is harmless.

- Saline implants are available with smooth-walled or textured (more expensive) surfaces.

- Saline implants do not feel as natural as silicone gel implants and are *not* guaranteed to last a lifetime.

- Numerous worldwide studies have consistently shown no link between silicone gel implants and any illness or disease. However, this does not discount the complaints or concerns of women who have questions about the safety of silicone implants.

- You should still be able to breast-feed after breast implantation unless silicone implants have been placed—antibodies to silicone are found in breast milk.

- Implants should not hinder breast self-examination unless there is extreme scarring around the implant.

- Breast implants *can* obscure mammograms.

- It is extremely important to notify your mammography technologist of the presence of breast implants; additional views are necessary and special care needs to be taken to minimize the possibility of rupture.

- Research is ongoing to develop a more natural-feeling and safe implant that also will not obscure mammograms. Clinical studies are evaluating soy implants. Soy implants have a more natural feel; however, there is a "soy" odor.

Procedure

Since the 1950s, over two million American women have had their breasts augmented, and the procedure has a very high satisfaction rate. You must make many important decisions if you choose this procedure—the location of the incisions; whether to place the implant over or under the muscle; and the type, size, texture, and shape of the implants. Be as well informed as possible so that you can be a part of this decision-making process. The surgical options you choose may be determining factors in your physician selection. Remember that different doctors use different techniques and usually recommend the one(s) in which they are trained and experienced. You and your physician must take into consideration your lifestyle, your body type, the types of clothes you wear, and your desired look. In general, if you undergo a breast augmentation, here's what you can expect.

ANESTHESIA

Breast augmentation is usually performed under general anesthesia, but some doctors perform it under intravenous sedation with local anesthesia. The type of anesthesia is dependent on the procedure to be performed, the doctor's choice, and the patient's medical history or desires.

INCISIONS

With saline implants, the incisions are just over an inch long because the implants are inflated *after* insertion. A larger incision is necessary for silicone implants because they are inserted in their inflated state. Additionally, there are four possible locations for the incisions.

Inframammary—in the crease underneath the breast. This scar is not visible unless you are lying down.

Circumareolar—on the lower edge of the areola.

Axillary—in the underarm. The incision is larger and can be seen when you raise your arm. The implant is placed with the aid of an endoscope.

STEPS IN THE BREAST AUGMENTATION PROCEDURE

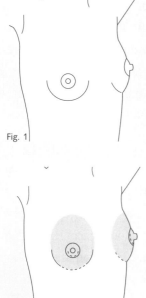

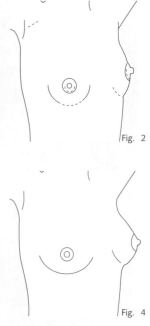

Fig. 1

Fig. 2

Fig. 3

Fig. 4

Breast augmentation is performed to increase the size of the breasts or to correct a difference in size between the breasts (Figure 1).

Incisions can be made in one of four places (Figure 2): under the arm, in the crease under the breast, in the bottom half of the areola, or in the navel (not shown).

In Figure 3, the shaded areas indicate pockets that are created to allow for the implants.

Figure 4 shows breasts that appear fuller and/or more even in size.

Umbilical—in the navel. Implant placement is aided with an endoscope. Only a few doctors are trained in this technique. Implants can only be placed above the muscle with this technique.

The choice should be determined by you and your physician. If a physician recommends a location that you are not comfortable with, ask him if he is experienced with the technique you want. If he is not, you may want to choose another physician. Whichever type of incision is used, the breast tissue is then lifted up and a pocket for the implant is created either under or above the breast (pectoral) muscle.

TYPES OF IMPLANTS

A number of different types of breast implants are available. They vary in fill material, shape, and texture. You and your doctor will discuss the shape and size (measured in cubic centimeters) that will best achieve your desired look. Some women want a more rounded look and others a more natural look. Some physicians choose to use only round implants and feel that they can accomplish a natural look by placing the implants under the muscle. Each physician may also have a different opinion regarding smooth versus textured implants.

Most physicians recommend the shape and/or texture in which they have training or experience. Discuss all of these aspects at length with your physician and ask him what has determined his recommendations. Your physician selection may be dependent upon your comfort level with his recommendations. These are the types of implants you and your doctor will discuss:

Silicone

Silicone gel implants are available only to certain patients: those who already have them in place, those who have had repeated problems with saline implants, those who have had a mastectomy (breast removal), those who have severe ptosis (drooping) of the breast(s) requiring a mastopexy (breast lift), or those who have specific medical or surgical deformities. If you choose silicone gel implants, you must be a part of a clinical study and must go to a physician who is approved to place silicone implants. The implants are made of a solid silicone elastomer shell and are available with either smooth or textured surfaces. Silicone implants require a larger incision because they are inserted prefilled.

Saline

These implants are inserted *before* inflation so that there is a smaller incision. This is the implant to choose if you want to be able to breast-feed after implantation. Available in smooth and textured surfaces, the shell is an elastomer of silicone.

Shapes

Implants are also available in different shapes: round and teardrop.

Texture

Implants are available with smooth and textured surfaces. Some physicians feel that the tissues may adhere better to the textured surface. However, the smooth implants are less expensive.

There is no guarantee that your implants will last a lifetime. When considering this procedure, it is important that you feel comfortable with the fact that you may need new implants sometime during your lifetime. Obviously, this will involve another surgery with the associated costs, i.e., physician, facility, anesthesiologist, and implant fees (if not covered by the manufacturer).

IMPLANT PLACEMENT

The implant can be placed above or beneath the pectoral muscle; each position has its own advantages. You and your doctor must consider your desired look, your lifestyle, and the amount of existing breast tissue. For example, a physician may recommend placement over the muscle for a woman who has a large amount of breast tissue or for a woman who has a very developed pectoral muscle. In both cases, the implants may not show if they are placed under the muscle. However, if a muscular woman is a kick boxer, the physician may recommend placement under the muscle to avoid possible rupture if she were hit in the chest area. Implants placed under the muscle may require a longer recuperation period.

Breast cancer may be harder to detect in the future when the implant is placed above the muscle. This is an important consideration. Also, when the implant is placed above the muscle, some women can hear the saline "slosh" when they move vigorously.

SUTURES AND RESTRICTIVE GARMENTS

The incisions are closed with sutures (which may or may not be dissolvable), and while you are still in the operating room, a restrictive bra may be placed on you. This holds the implants in place and aids the skin in adhering to the underlying tissue. It also helps to reduce swelling.

LENGTH OF SURGICAL PROCEDURE

Breast augmentation should take approximately one and one-half to two and one-half hours.

Prior to Surgery

Before surgery, you and your doctor will first make several important decisions. Then you will prepare for surgery and be given prescriptions and instructions. The following sections will give you an overview of the process.

ASSESSMENT

Bring pictures from magazines showing your desired look. Also, bring a full-cup bra in your desired cup size. Your physician should discuss with you what you want to accomplish and should assess the size of your breasts in relation and proportion to the rest of your body. Different-sized implants (measured in cubic centimeters) may be placed in the cups so that you and the physician can determine the best size for you. Depending on the laxity of the tissue and the size of your breasts, your physician may recommend a breast reduction and/or a breast lift in conjunction with implants. The implants alone may not be sufficient to achieve your desired look. This may be the case if your breasts are different sizes. Be absolutely clear and in agreement with your doctor about what look and size you want for your breasts.

LOCATION OF INCISIONS AND TYPE AND SIZE OF IMPLANTS

Decide with your physician on the location of the incisions, the type of implants (silicone or saline, smooth or textured), the size and shape of the implants, and their placement (above or beneath the pectoral muscle).

PREOPERATIVE VISIT

You should be instructed to have certain lab tests, i.e., blood work, chest x-ray, EKG. You may go to your family doctor, an independent lab, or a hospital facility. The physician you have chosen may arrange for the performance of these tests. You may also be instructed to have a mammogram if you have not had one recently.

You may sign all of your surgical consent forms, and be given pre- and post-operative instructions at this time. You should also be given your prescriptions for before and after surgery. Make sure that everything you and your physician have agreed on, such as implant size, is stated on the consent form.

PRESCRIPTIONS

Some or all of these may be prescribed, in addition to others not listed.

- multivitamins—to be taken ten days to two weeks before and after surgery
- vitamin C—500 milligrams twice daily, to be taken ten days to two weeks before and after surgery
- vitamin E cream
- pain medication
- antinausea medication
- oral antibiotics—it's extremely important to take all of the antibiotics that are prescribed (the implant is sterile, but a foreign material is being placed in your body)
- sleeping medication

    Be sure to follow your doctor's instructions.

PRE- AND POSTOPERATIVE INSTRUCTIONS

These suggestions are intended to make you more comfortable and help you heal. To learn more, turn to the section on recovery in this chapter. Your doctor may have different or additional instructions. Follow them to the letter.

- Stop smoking, discontinue the use of alcohol, and stop taking vitamin E and any medications containing aspirin or ibuprofen (two weeks pre- and postoperative is usually recommended). Check with your doctor regarding any other medications (including homeopathic/herbal products) that you are currently taking.
- Be sure you understand how and when to take your prescriptions.
- Know how to cleanse the surgical areas the night before or the morning of your surgery.
- Do not have food (including gum or mints) or drink (including water) for a minimum of six to eight hours prior to surgery. (Follow your surgical facility's preoperative instructions.)

- Have someone drive you to and from surgery.
- Have someone stay with you the first night after surgery (the first twenty-four to forty-eight hours, optimally).
- Do not lift anything heavier than a small telephone book for at least ten days.
- If you blow-dry your hair, it may be more comfortable to keep the dryer at a low angle for ten days to two weeks.
- Do not drive for a week to ten days after surgery and while taking pain medication.
- The procedure may require that a supportive bra, which may be provided, be worn for four to six weeks after surgery. You may want to purchase a second garment to wear while you launder the other. Some physicians use Ace wraps to prevent the implants from riding up. Do not wear an underwire bra, especially if the incisions are in the crease underneath the breast.
- Your doctor may instruct you to apply cold compresses, usually for twenty minutes every hour for a minimum of forty-eight hours. Do *not* apply cold compresses to the nipple area.
- You must sleep on your back with your upper body elevated for at least the first week to ten days.
- Do not expose the breasts to the sun or tanning beds, especially while bruising is visible, because the pigmentation of the skin may change permanently. Optimally, sun and tanning beds should be avoided completely for skin care and health.
- Restrict upper-body activity for four to six weeks.
- Avoid aerobic activity for a minimum of three to four weeks after surgery.

Recovery

Everyone heals differently. Healing is affected by your genetics, your physical and emotional well-being, whether you smoke and/or drink alcohol, your pain tolerance, the extent of the surgery, and how well you follow the doctor's instructions. The initial healing period for breast augmentation can take, on an average, from four days to one week. If the implants have been placed below the muscle, it may take seven to ten days.

FIRST DAY POSTOPERATIVE

You may want to sleep the first day after surgery. You will experience some level of soreness and tenderness in the breast area and will need help getting in and out of bed for the first few days.

SWELLING AND BRUISING

You can expect some swelling and bruising after surgery. This usually clears up in two to three weeks. Keep in mind that the body does not heal symmetrically.

By the third week, you should still have some minor swelling, which can last for months (as long as six to nine). The bruising may be gone by the third week but could possibly last for six weeks.

NUMBNESS AND ITCHING

You may have some temporary numbness, which should dissipate in a maximum of six months. If the incision sites itch, gently rub the areas—do not scratch them. Ask your doctor if you can apply cream or ointment to relieve the itching, and only use what is recommended.

COMPRESSION GARMENT/DRESSING

A restrictive bra may be placed on you while you are still in the operating room; some physicians use wraps. Your doctor should give you full instructions concerning the length of time this garment or wrap is to be worn. Many patients feel more comfortable with it on and choose to wear it longer than their doctors require.

COLD COMPRESSES

Cold compresses applied to the chest area may relieve some of the discomfort and can greatly reduce the swelling. These should be applied every hour for twenty minutes for a minimum of forty-eight hours (some doctors recommend seventy-two hours) after surgery. Ice should never be placed directly on the skin. Either use cold compresses or place a cloth between the ice bag and your skin. In some cases, your doctor may have instructed you *not* to use cold compresses. Follow your doctor's instructions. Do *not* apply cold compresses to the nipple area because the cold restricts blood flow.

BODY POSITION

Sleep on your back with your upper body elevated for at least the first week to ten days.

WALKING/EXERCISE

By the third day, you may be allowed to start walking around the house. Many patients say that the third day is the most uncomfortable, so do not overdo it—listen to your body. If you feel tired, rest. Do not try to raise your arms. By the fourth day, you can possibly resume a light routine—no strenuous activity or lifting. Most physicians recommend that you wait a minimum of three to four weeks to resume aerobic exercise.

MASSAGE

Some physicians recommend massage to keep the breasts soft and/or a postoperative vitamin E cream may be recommended to lessen capsule formation. Follow your doctor's instructions.

SUTURES

The sutures should be removed (if they were not dissolvable) at your first postoperative appointment, at about one week.

INCISION LINES

You should receive instructions on the care of your incisions and when you can bathe. Your scars may remain red for four to six weeks and should gradually fade. Most scars become barely noticeable over time.

Pain

As with recovery times, pain tolerance is different for everyone. What one person may consider pain, another person may consider discomfort.

LEVEL OF PAIN/DISCOMFORT

Generally, with breast augmentation, if the implant is placed above the muscle, there is minimal discomfort during the postoperative period. The discomfort may be more pronounced if the implant is placed beneath the muscle.

PAIN MEDICATION

Most discomfort can be controlled with pain medications you have been prescribed or Extra Strength Tylenol. You may find it necessary to take pain medication for the first three to four days.

Risks/Complications

Although problems are unlikely, you need to be aware of what can happen and what action you should take. Most risks/complications will be avoided if you make an informed decision, choose a qualified physician, and follow your physician's instructions.

BLEEDING

Call your doctor immediately if there is any bleeding from the incisions.

INFECTION

Antibiotics are given to you intravenously during the procedure, and you may be instructed to take an oral antibiotic after surgery. Follow your doctor's instructions.

HEMATOMA

A hematoma, a collection of blood or fluid beneath the skin, is unlikely. However, if it does occur, it can be treated with a compression garment. Occasionally, surgery may be required.

ASYMMETRY

This problem may require another surgery.

IRREGULARITIES

Rippling of the implant edges is less likely if the implant is placed beneath the muscle and the implant is filled to the manufacturer's specifications.

CAPSULAR CONTRACTURE

The body attempts to "wall off" the implant by forming a fibrous capsule around it. The thickness of the capsule formed varies from patient to patient and is influenced by heredity or the presence of postoperative hematoma or infection. Depending on the severity of the capsule, it may be broken up manually by the physician or it may require removal and/or implant replacement.

CHANGES IN NIPPLE SENSATION

Nipple sensation may increase or decrease after breast augmentation. This change may or may not be permanent.

HYPERTROPHIC SCARRING

Report any signs immediately to your doctor; this scarring can be treated if caught early. (See "Definitions of Scarring/Skin Changes," page 56.)

HYPERPIGMENTED SCARRING

This scarring can be cosmetically tattooed. (See "Definitions of Scarring/Skin Changes," page 56.)

$\mathcal{B}$reast Lift–Mastopexy

A breast lift is a procedure designed to restore a more youthful appearance to sagging breasts.

As we age, breast tissue loses some of its elasticity and fat. Many women's breasts droop after pregnancy and/or breast-feeding. Additionally, a significant weight gain and subsequent loss of weight can result in sagging breasts because the skin has been stretched. Women who make the decision to have a mastopexy are usually very satisfied with the results. However, as with any surgical procedure, it is very important to be informed. Here are some interesting facts about mastopexy.

- Women who go braless tend to have droopier breasts; gravity plays a part in causing breasts to sag.

- Mastopexy lifts the nipple to the level of the crease underneath your breasts.

- A breast lift changes the shape of the breast, not the volume.

- This procedure can be performed in conjunction with a breast augmentation if you feel you do not have adequate breast tissue.

- Upon removal of breast implants, a breast lift may sometimes be necessary.

- This procedure is not recommended for smokers.

- Remember—time marches on. The effects of aging and gravity will not stop after surgery. The more you wear a bra (optimally twenty-four hours a day), the less your breast tissue will stretch.

Procedure

Many women choose to have a mastopexy performed because most conventional bras are not enough to support their breasts and/or they don't like the way their breasts look. A breast lift can leave a moderately noticeable scar (depending on the technique used), but patients are willing to accept a scar so that they will look better in their clothes. Remember that different doctors use different techniques and usually recommend the one(s) in which they are trained and experienced. Educate yourself so that you can be a part of this decision-making process. In general, if you undergo a mastopexy, here's what you can expect.

ANESTHESIA

A breast lift (mastopexy) is usually performed under general anesthesia, but some doctors perform it under intravenous sedation with local anesthesia. The type of anesthesia is dependent on the procedure to be performed, the doctor's choice, and the patient's medical history or desires.

TECHNIQUES

The technique used will depend on the amount of ptosis (drooping) of the breast and your physician's training and experience. The location of the incisions is dictated by the technique used. The following techniques are most often used for breast lifts:

Crescent—for mild ptosis. This is an upper-areolar incision only.

Circumareolar—for mild ptosis. One continuous incision around the areola can be used.

Vertical—for moderate ptosis. The same continuous incision around the areola is used, along with a vertical incision down the lower half of the breast to the chest wall.

Anchor or inverted T (the most common technique used)—for severe ptosis. The same continuous incision around the areola with the vertical incision is used, along with a five- to seven-inch incision made in the crease underneath the breast.

NIPPLE AND AREOLA

Most surgeons do not completely detach the nipple. It is freed via the circumareolar incision, but attachment to the tissue, which includes milk ducts, blood supply, and nerve endings, is maintained. However, nipple sensation and the ability to breast-feed may still be lost.

STEPS IN THE BREAST LIFT PROCEDURE

The location of the incisions is dictated by the technique used, and upon the amount of the ptosis (drooping).

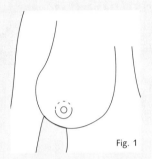

Fig. 1

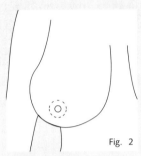

Fig. 2

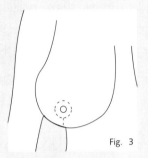

Fig. 3

Crescent: For mild ptosis. Upper areolar incision only (Figure 1).

Circumareolar: For mild ptosis. One continuous incision around the areola (Figure 2).

Vertical: For moderate ptosis. The same continuous incision around the areola is used, along with a vertical incision down the lower half of the breast to the chest wall (Figure 3).

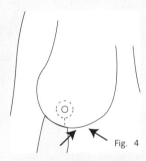

Fig. 4

Anchor or Inverted "T": The most common technique used for severe ptosis. The same continuous incision around the areola with the vertical incision is used, along with a five- to seven-inch incision made in the crease underneath the breast (Figure 4).

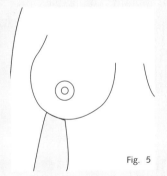

Fig. 5

The breast lift procedure chages the shape of the breast (Figure 5).

With all techniques, excess skin is cut away so that the remaining skin is tightened. At this point, if you have chosen to have breast implants in conjunction with the breast lift, the implants are placed, usually underneath the muscle. (See "Breast Augmentation," page 87.) The areola is then repositioned.

The tissue underneath the skin is sutured with dissolvable stitches, and drains may be placed. The skin is then sutured.

COMPRESSION GARMENTS/DRESSING

While you are still in the operating room, a restrictive bra or dressing should be placed on you. This provides support and aids the skin in adhering to the underlying tissue. It also helps reduce swelling.

LENGTH OF PROCEDURE

A breast lift should take approximately two to four hours.

Prior to Surgery

Before surgery, you and your doctor will first make several important decisions. Then you will prepare for surgery and be given prescriptions and instructions. The following sections will give you an overview of the process.

ASSESSMENT

Depending on the size and laxity of your breasts, your physician may recommend a breast reduction and/or implants in conjunction with a breast lift. (See "Breast Augmentation," page 87.) Be absolutely clear and in agreement with your doctor about the look and size you want for your breasts. Discuss with your physician the location of the incisions.

Note: Many doctors may choose not to perform a breast lift on smokers. Smoking diminishes blood flow and may result in the breast skin and nipples not surviving the surgery. Scars would then replace this dead tissue, potentially causing severe disfigurement.

PREOPERATIVE VISIT

You should be instructed to have certain lab tests, i.e., blood work, chest x-ray, EKG. You may go to your family doctor, a hospital facility, or an independent lab. The physician you have chosen may arrange for the performance of these tests. You may also be instructed to have a mammogram if you have not had one recently.

You may sign all of your surgical consent forms, and be given pre- and postoperative instructions at this time. You should also be given your prescriptions for before and after surgery. Make sure that everything you and your physician have agreed on is stated on the consent form.

PRESCRIPTIONS

Some or all of these may be prescribed, in addition to others not listed.

- multivitamins—to be taken ten days to two weeks before and after surgery

- vitamin C—500 milligrams twice daily, to be taken ten days to two weeks before and after surgery

- vitamin E cream

- pain medication

- antinausea medication

- oral antibiotics

- sleeping medication

  Be sure to follow your doctor's instructions.

PRE- AND POSTOPERATIVE INSTRUCTIONS

These suggestions are intended to make you more comfortable and help you heal. To learn more, turn to the section on recovery in this chapter. Your doctor may have different or additional instructions. Follow them to the letter.

- If you have regular mammograms or are over the age of forty, schedule a mammogram prior to your procedure and then again after the swelling and tenderness have disappeared completely (three to six months). In this way, the changes resulting from your surgery can be documented.

- Stop smoking (see note, page 102), discontinue the use of alcohol, and stop taking vitamin E and any medications containing aspirin or ibuprofen (two weeks pre- and postoperative is usually recommended). Check with your doctor regarding any other medications (including homeopathic/herbal products) that you are currently taking.

- Be sure you understand how and when to take your prescriptions.

- Know how to cleanse the surgical areas the night before or morning of your surgery.

- Do not have food (including gum or mints) or drink (including water) for a minimum of six to eight hours prior to surgery. (Follow your surgical facility's preoperative instructions.)

- Have someone drive you to and from surgery.

- Have someone stay with you the first night after surgery (the first twenty-four to forty-eight hours, optimally).

- Do not lift anything heavier than a small telephone book for at least ten days.

- If you blow-dry your hair, it may be more comfortable to keep the dryer at a low angle for ten days to two weeks.

- Do not drive for a week to ten days after surgery and while taking pain medication.

- The procedure may require that a supportive bra or dressing, which should be provided, be worn for four to six weeks after surgery. You may want to purchase a second garment to wear while you launder the other. Do not wear an underwire bra for six weeks, especially if the incisions are in the crease underneath the breast.

- If drains are placed, they will be removed in two to three days.

- Your doctor may instruct you to apply cold compresses, usually for twenty minutes every hour for a minimum of forty-eight hours. Do *not* apply cold compresses to the nipple area.

- You must sleep on your back with your upper body elevated for at least the first week to ten days.

- Do not lie face down for at least three weeks.

- Do not expose the breasts to the sun or tanning beds, especially while bruising is visible. (The pigmentation of the skin may change permanently.) Optimally, these should be avoided completely for skin care and health.

- Restrict upper-body activity for four to six weeks.

- Avoid aerobic activity for a minimum of three to four weeks after surgery.

Recovery

Everyone heals differently. Healing is affected by your genetics, your physical and emotional well-being, whether you smoke and/or drink alcohol, your pain tolerance, the extent of the surgery, and how well you follow the doctor's instructions. The initial healing period for a breast lift can take, on an average, from one to two weeks.

FIRST DAY POSTOPERATIVE

You may want to sleep the first day after surgery. You will experience some soreness and tenderness in the breast area and will need help getting in and out of bed for the first few days.

SWELLING AND BRUISING

After surgery, you can expect to experience some swelling and bruising, which usually clears up in two to three weeks. Keep in mind that the body does not heal symmetrically. By the third week, you may still have some minor swelling, which can last for as long as six to nine months. The bruising may be gone by the third week but could possibly last for six weeks.

NUMBNESS AND ITCHING

You may also have some temporary numbness, which should dissipate in a maximum of six months. Also, if the incision sites itch, gently rub the areas—do not scratch them. Ask your doctor if you can apply some cream or ointment to relieve the itching and only use what is recommended.

COMPRESSION GARMENT

A restrictive bra will probably have been placed on you while you were still in the operating room. Your doctor will give you full instructions concerning the length of time this garment is to be worn. Many patients feel more comfortable with it on and choose to wear it longer than their doctors require.

COLD COMPRESSES

Cold compresses applied to the chest area may relieve some of the discomfort and can greatly reduce the swelling. These should be applied every hour for twenty minutes for a minimum of forty-eight hours (some doctors recommend seventy-two hours) after surgery. Ice should never be placed directly on the skin or the nipples. Either use cold compresses or place a cloth between the ice bag and your skin. In some cases, your doctor may instruct you not to use cold compresses. Follow your doctor's instructions. Do *not* apply cold compresses to the nipple area.

BODY POSITION

Sleep on your back, with your upper body elevated, for at least the first week to ten days.

WALKING/EXERCISE

By the third day, you may be allowed to start walking around the house. Many patients say that the third day is the most uncomfortable, so do not overdo it—listen to your body.

If you feel tired, rest. Do not try to raise your arms. By the fourth day, you may be able to resume a light routine—no strenuous activity or lifting. Most physicians recommend that you wait a minimum of three to four weeks to resume aerobic exercise.

DRAINS

If drains were placed, these should be removed in two to three days. Removal of the drains may cause some discomfort, so consider taking your pain medication prior to this appointment.

INCISION LINES

You should receive instructions on the care of your incisions and when you can bathe. The sutures should be removed in seven to fourteen days. Your scars may remain red for four to six weeks and should gradually fade. Most scars become barely noticeable over time.

AGING AND GRAVITY

Remember—time marches on. The effects of aging and gravity will not stop after surgery. The more you wear a bra (optimally twenty-four hours a day), the less your breast tissue can stretch.

Pain

As with recovery times, pain tolerance is different for everyone. What one person may consider pain, another person may consider discomfort.

LEVEL OF PAIN/DISCOMFORT

Generally, with a breast lift there is minimal to moderate discomfort during the postoperative period.

PAIN MEDICATION

Most discomfort can be controlled with pain medications you have been prescribed or Extra Strength Tylenol. You may find it necessary to take pain medication for the first three to four days.

Risks/Complications

Although problems are unlikely, you need to be aware of what can happen and what action you should take. Most risks/complications will be avoided if you make an informed decision, choose a qualified physician, and follow your physician's instructions.

BLEEDING

Call your doctor immediately if there is any bleeding from the incisions.

INFECTION

Antibiotics are given to you intravenously during the procedure, and you will probably be instructed to take an oral antibiotic after surgery. Follow your doctor's instructions.

HEMATOMA

A hematoma, a collection of blood or fluid beneath the skin, is unlikely. However, if it does occur, it can be treated by drainage with a needle or with a compression garment.

ASYMMETRY

This problem may require another surgery.

CHANGES IN NIPPLE SENSATION

Nipple sensation may increase or decrease after a breast lift. This change may or may not be permanent.

HYPERTROPHIC SCARRING

Report any signs immediately to your doctor; this scarring can be treated if caught early. (See "Definitions of Scarring/Skin Changes," page 56.)

HYPERPIGMENTED SCARRING

This scarring can be cosmetically tattooed. (See "Definitions of Scarring/Skin Changes," page 56.)

CAPSULAR CONTRACTURE (IF IMPLANTS ARE USED)

The body attempts to "wall off" the implant by forming a fibrous capsule around it. The thickness of the capsule formed varies from patient to patient and is influenced by heredity or the presence of postoperative hematoma or infection. Depending on the severity of the capsule, it may be able to be broken up manually by the physician or it may require removal and/or implant replacement.

$\mathcal{B}$reast Reconstruction

$\mathbf{B}$reast reconstruction is performed to reconstruct the breast after breast cancer.

There are many factors for you to discuss with your plastic surgeon and oncologist when determining the timing and type of breast reconstruction to be performed. It may or may not take place at the same time as the mastectomy. However, the elimination of the breast cancer is your primary concern—it must take precedence over any considerations for reconstruction. You will be faced with a large number of decisions so it is extremely important for you to be totally informed. The following section will help you sort through some of the information that you will be presented. Here are some interesting facts about breast reconstruction.

- The reconstructive patient must have realistic expectations—the goal is to improve appearance, not attain perfection.

- Reconstruction at the same time as the mastectomy can be an emotional advantage for the patient.

- Some surgeons feel that it is advantageous to perform reconstructive surgery approximately three months after the mastectomy, to give the tissues time to heal and soften. However, many physicians feel that this is an antiquated view.

- Reconstruction of the areola and nipple, if desired, is usually performed in a separate surgery.

- Your surgeon may suggest completion of any chemotherapy or radiation therapies (if necessary) prior to any reconstructive surgery for locally advanced breast cancer.

Procedure

You and your physician must make many important decisions—whether the reconstruction will be performed at the same time as or after the mastectomy; the technique to be used; if implants are to be placed, whether they will be used for both breasts; and the fill material, size, shape, and texture of the implants. Remember that different doctors use different techniques and usually recommend the one(s) in which they are trained and experienced. Educate yourself so that you can be a part of this decision-making process. Your choices may even be a part of the determining factor in your choice of physician. In general, if you undergo breast reconstruction, here's what you can expect.

ANESTHESIA

Breast reconstruction is usually performed under general anesthesia. The type of anesthesia is dependent on the procedure to be performed, the doctor's choice, and the patient's medical history or desires.

INCISIONS

Placement of incisions depends on the location of the incisions used by the breast oncologic surgeon to remove breast tissue. The incisions may or may not be placed in the old incision sites.

TECHNIQUES

Many techniques are available. Which technique is used depends on the patient's desires, the physician's training and experience, the patient's health and anatomy, the amount of tissue available, and the other breast's appearance. The following are the most common reconstructive techniques:

Breast Implant

If there is sufficient tissue (skin), a silicone or saline implant may be placed beneath the pectoral muscle. (See "Breast Augmentation," page 87.) Most often, a tissue expander is necessary prior to implant placement.

Tissue Expander

This balloon-like device with a reservoir is placed under the pectoral muscle during the original surgery. Over a period of a number of weeks, sterile saline is injected into the reservoir, gradually stretching the skin. Some expanders can be left in to serve as an implant; other expanders must be removed and replaced with an implant after the skin and muscle are expanded.

Tram Flap

A large flap of lower abdominal skin and fat, along with a part of one or both of the rectus abdominis muscles, is either rotated through the abdomen or separated and reattached to the chest wall and shaped. (See "Tummy Tuck—Abdominoplasty," page 245.) The major advantage of this procedure is that there is no need for an implant because of the abundance of tissue available. The patient also benefits by getting a "tummy tuck." However, this is a major procedure, which can require four to six days in the hospital. This procedure is not recommended for patients who do not have excess abdominal fat.

Latissimus Dorsi Flap

A portion of this broad muscle in the back, along with overlying skin and fat, is rotated around the side to the chest wall and shaped. Since there is usually insufficient tissue to completely reconstruct the breast, an implant may be necessary.

Free-Flap Transfer

Tissue from the abdomen, buttocks, hips, or thighs, along with the blood vessels, is completely removed and transplanted to the chest wall. The blood vessels are joined to the blood vessels in the armpit.

Nipple and Areola Reconstruction

Reconstruction of the nipple and areola are usually performed in a separate surgery once the reconstructed breast has healed. The nipple can be more accurately positioned in this manner. Local tissue from the breast reconstruction, abdomen, and/or groin (labia) may be used. If desired, cosmetic tattooing can be performed later to match the color of the nipple to the other breast.

Prior to Surgery

Your primary concern is to eliminate the breast cancer. However, you need to be aware of your options for reconstruction, as some techniques may or may not take place at the same time as the mastectomy. As with all cosmetic or reconstructive surgery, the goal is to improve appearance, not attain perfection. Be absolutely clear and in agreement with your physician.

Many factors can affect the recovery, pain, risks, and complications associated with breast reconstruction. Among these are the technique used, the therapy utilized to treat the cancer, and whether the procedure is performed at the same time as the mastectomy or afterwards.

Once you and your physician have decided which technique is best for you, turn to the sections that describe and will guide you through these procedures in detail. (See "Breast Augmentation," page 87 and "Tummy Tuck—Abdominoplasty," page 245.)

STEPS IN THE BREAST RECONSTRUCTION PROCEDURE

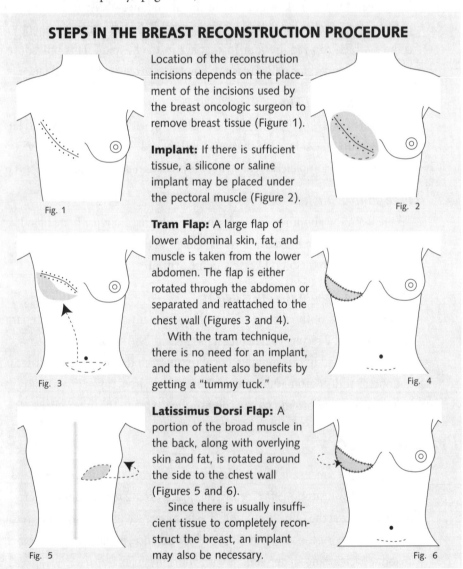

Location of the reconstruction incisions depends on the placement of the incisions used by the breast oncologic surgeon to remove breast tissue (Figure 1).

Implant: If there is sufficient tissue, a silicone or saline implant may be placed under the pectoral muscle (Figure 2).

Fig. 1

Fig. 2

Tram Flap: A large flap of lower abdominal skin, fat, and muscle is taken from the lower abdomen. The flap is either rotated through the abdomen or separated and reattached to the chest wall (Figures 3 and 4).

With the tram technique, there is no need for an implant, and the patient also benefits by getting a "tummy tuck."

Fig. 3

Fig. 4

Latissimus Dorsi Flap: A portion of the broad muscle in the back, along with overlying skin and fat, is rotated around the side to the chest wall (Figures 5 and 6).

Since there is usually insufficient tissue to completely reconstruct the breast, an implant may also be necessary.

Fig. 5

Fig. 6

$\mathcal{B}$reast Reduction for Men (Gynecomastia)

$\mathbf{B}$reast reduction for enlarged male breasts (gynecomastia) may be desired for cosmetic and/or emotional reasons.

Some men develop overly large breasts; this condition is called gynecomastia. This condition may result from certain medications, such as digitalis or Tagamet. Additionally, it may be caused by a hormone imbalance, a large amount of body fat, or tumors. It is also associated with the use of marijuana. Many men have been self-conscious all of their lives about this condition and consequently have not become informed about the different techniques available to address it. The following section will help you sort through the options. Here are some interesting facts about gynecomastia.

- There should be a very thorough exam of the patient's breasts, body fat content, and medical history to determine the proper treatment.

- A number of different techniques are used to reduce enlarged male breasts including liposuction, surgical removal of excess breast tissue (breast reduction), and mastopexy (breast lift), which reduces the breast tissue and lifts the level of the nipple.

- A breast reduction changes the volume and shape of the breast; a breast lift changes the shape of the breast.

- The areola (nipple) may have to be repositioned because large breasts most often are "ptotic" (sagging).

- Some physicians who perform male breast reductions may recommend a mammogram prior to a patient's procedure to determine that there is no breast cancer present. This would depend on the age of the patient and his medical history.

• This procedure is not recommended for smokers.

Once you and your physician have decided which technique is best for you, turn to the sections that describe and will guide you through these procedures in detail. (See "Liposuction," page 217; "Breast Lift," page 99; and "Breast Reduction," page 115.)

Breast Reduction–Mammaplasty

Breast reduction is performed to reduce the size of the breasts. It may be desired for cosmetic, emotional, and/or physical reasons.

Many women do not like how they look in their clothes because of their excessively large breasts. Excessively large breasts can cause physical problems such as back and/or neck pain, poor posture, notches in the shoulders caused by bra straps digging into them, and rashes and/or infections underneath the breasts. Additionally, the psychological concerns surrounding large breasts make breast reduction a highly sought procedure. Breast reduction is one of the few cosmetic surgery procedures that is performed on teenagers (once their breasts have completed development). This procedure carries a very high satisfaction rate for patients of all ages. As with all surgical procedures, it is important to be informed. Here are some interesting facts about mammaplasty.

- This procedure reduces the breast tissue and lifts the nipple to the level of the crease underneath the breast.

- A breast reduction changes the volume and shape of the breast and the size of the areola, if desired.

- The areola usually has to be repositioned because large breasts most often are "ptotic" (sagging).

- Remember—time marches on. The effects of aging and gravity will not stop after surgery. The more you wear a bra (optimally twenty-four hours a day), the less your breast tissue will stretch.

- It is recommended that smokers stop smoking fourteen days prior to surgery. Some physicians do not recommend this procedure for smokers.

Procedures

The most important decision you must make is the breast size that you want upon completion of this procedure. You and your physician must take into consideration your lifestyle, your body type, the types of clothes you wear, and your desired look. A mammaplasty can leave noticeable scars, but patients are willing to accept them so that they will look better in their clothes. Educate yourself so that you can be a part of this decision-making process. Remember that different doctors use different techniques and usually recommend the one(s) in which they are trained and experienced. In general, if you undergo a mammaplasty, here's what you can expect.

ANESTHESIA

Breast reduction is usually performed under general anesthesia. However, the type of anesthesia used is dependent on the procedure to be performed, the doctor's choice, and the patient's medical history or desires.

TECHNIQUE

While you are upright, your breasts should be very precisely marked with a permanent marker. The anesthesia will then be administered. The surgeon makes a continuous incision around the areola, with a vertical incision below it (known as an "inverted keyhole incision"), connected to a horizontal incision made in the crease underneath the breast. This last incision is usually the whole width of the breast.

Most surgeons do not completely detach the nipple. It is freed via the circumareolar incision, but attachment to the tissue (which includes milk ducts, blood supply, and nerve endings) is maintained.

Excess breast tissue, fat, and skin are removed above, below, and on either side of the nipple. Some surgeons use liposuction to remove fatty breast tissue in the underarm area. The areola may or may not be reduced and is then repositioned and sutured into place.

The tissue and skin on both sides of the breasts are brought together and sutured (some physicians use only dissolvable sutures; some use a combination of dissolvable and nondissolvable). Drains may be placed.

STEPS IN THE BREAST REDUCTION PROCEDURE

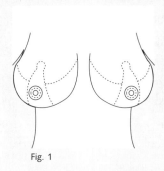

Fig. 1

A continuous incision around the areola is made with a vertical incision below it, connected to a horizontal incision in the crease underneath the breast (usually the whole width of the breast) (Figure 1).

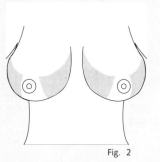

Fig. 2

Excess breast tissue, fat, and skin are removed (Figure 2).

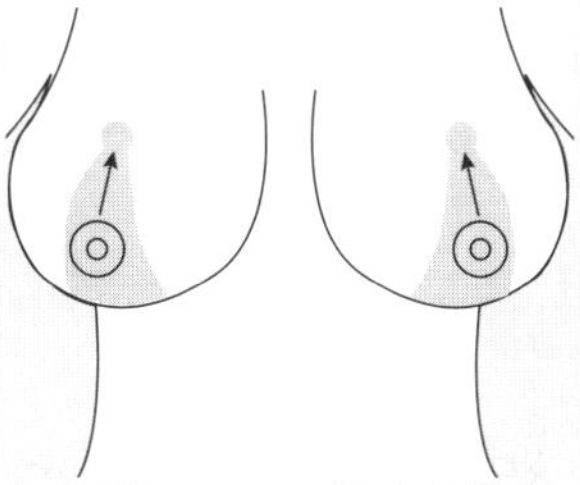

The nipple, which has been "freed up" via the circumareolar incision, is placed in its new position (Figure 3).

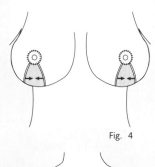

Fig. 3

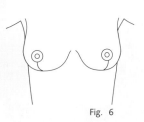

Fig. 4

The tissue and skin on both sides of the breast are brought together (Figure 4).

All of the incision lines are sutured and drains may be placed (Figure 5).

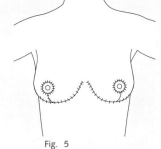

Fig. 5

This procedure changes the volume and shape of the breast and the size of the areola, if desired (Figure 6).

Fig. 6

COMPRESSION GARMENT/DRESSING

While you are still in the operating room, a restrictive bra or dressing should be placed on you. This provides support and aids the skin in adhering to the underlying tissue. It also helps reduce swelling.

LENGTH OF PROCEDURE

A breast reduction will take approximately three to five hours.

Prior to Surgery

Before surgery, you and your doctor will first make several important decisions. Then you will prepare for surgery and be given prescriptions and instructions. The following sections will give you an overview of the process.

ASSESSMENT

Bring pictures from magazines of your desired look. Your physician should assess the size and laxity (degree of sagging) of your breasts. Be absolutely clear and in agreement with your doctor about what look and size you want for your breasts. Discuss with your physician the location of the incisions.

Note: Many doctors may choose not to perform a breast reduction on smokers. Smoking diminishes blood flow and may result in the breast skin and nipples not surviving the surgery. Scars would then replace this dead tissue, potentially causing severe disfigurement.

PREOPERATIVE VISIT

You should be instructed to have certain lab tests, i.e., blood work, chest x-ray, EKG. You may go to your family doctor, a hospital facility, or an independent lab. The physician you have chosen may arrange for the performance of these tests. You should also be instructed to have a mammogram if you have not had one recently.

You may sign all of your surgical consent forms and be given pre- and postoperative instructions at this time. You should also be given your prescriptions for before and after surgery. Make sure that everything you and your physician have agreed on, such as breast size, is stated on the consent form.

PRESCRIPTIONS

Some or all of these may be prescribed, in addition to others not listed:

- multivitamins—to be taken ten days to two weeks before and after surgery
- vitamin C—500 milligrams twice daily, to be taken ten days to two weeks before and after surgery
- vitamin E cream
- pain medication

- antinausea medication
- oral antibiotics
- sleeping medication

Be sure to follow your doctor's instructions.

PRE- AND POSTOPERATIVE INSTRUCTIONS

These suggestions are intended to make you more comfortable and help you heal. To learn more, turn to the section on recovery in this chapter. Your doctor may have different or additional instructions. Follow them to the letter.

- If you have regular mammograms or are over the age of forty, schedule a mammogram prior to your procedure, and then again after the swelling and tenderness have disappeared completely (three to six months). In this way, the changes from your surgery can be documented.

- Stop smoking (see note, page 118), discontinue the use of alcohol, and stop taking vitamin E and any medications containing aspirin or ibuprofen (two weeks pre- and postoperative is usually recommended). Check with your doctor regarding any other medications (including homeopathic/herbal products) that you are currently taking.

- Be sure you understand how and when to take your prescriptions.

- Know how to cleanse the surgical areas the night before or morning of your surgery.

- Do not have food (including gum or mints) or drink (including water) for a minimum of six to eight hours prior to surgery. (Follow your surgical facility's preoperative instructions.)

- Have someone drive you to and from surgery.

- Have someone stay with you the first night after surgery (the first twenty-four to forty-eight hours, optimally). Some patients may require a one- to two-night stay in a hospital or overnight facility.

- Do not lift anything heavier than a small telephone book for at least ten days.

- If you blow-dry your hair, it may be more comfortable to keep the dryer at a low angle for ten days to two weeks.

- Do not drive for a week to ten days after surgery and while taking pain medication.

- The procedure requires that a supportive bra or dressing, which should be provided, be worn for four to six weeks after surgery. You may want to purchase a second garment to wear while you launder the other. Do not wear an underwire bra for six weeks.

- Your doctor may instruct you to apply cold compresses for twenty minutes every hour for a minimum of forty-eight hours. Do *not* apply cold compresses to the nipple area.

- You must sleep on your back, with your upper body elevated, for at least the first week to ten days.

- Do not lie face down for at least three weeks.

- Do not expose the breasts to the sun and tanning beds, especially while bruising is visible. (The pigmentation of the skin may change permanently.) Optimally, these should be avoided completely for skin care and health.

- Restrict upper-body activity for four to six weeks.

- Avoid aerobic activity for a minimum of three to four weeks after surgery.

Recovery

Everyone heals differently. Healing is affected by your genetics, your physical and emotional well-being, whether you smoke and/or drink alcohol, your pain tolerance, the extent of the surgery, and how well you follow the doctor's instructions. The initial healing period for a breast reduction can take, on an average, from one to two weeks.

FIRST DAY POSTOPERATIVE

You may want to sleep the first day after surgery. You will probably experience soreness and tenderness in the breast area and will need help getting in and out of bed for the first few days.

SWELLING AND BRUISING

After surgery, you can expect to experience some swelling and bruising, which usually clears up in two to three weeks. Keep in mind that the body does not heal symmetrically.

By the third week, you could still have some minor swelling, which can last for as long as six to nine months. The bruising may be gone by the third week but could possibly last for six weeks.

NUMBNESS AND ITCHING

You may also have some temporary numbness, which should dissipate in a maximum of six months. If the incision sites itch, gently rub the areas—do not scratch them. Ask your doctor if you can apply some cream or ointment to relieve the itching and only use what is recommended.

COMPRESSION GARMENT/DRESSING

A restrictive bra should have been placed on you while you were still in the operating room. Your doctor should give you full instructions concerning the length of time this garment is to be worn. Many patients feel more comfortable with it on and choose to wear it longer than the doctor requires.

COLD COMPRESSES

Cold compresses applied to the chest area may relieve some of the discomfort and can greatly reduce the swelling. These should be applied every hour for twenty minutes for a minimum of forty-eight hours (some doctors recommend seventy-two hours) after surgery. Ice should never be placed directly on the skin. Either use cold compresses or place a cloth between the ice bag and your skin. In some cases, your doctor may instruct you *not* to use cold compresses. Follow your doctor's instructions. Do *not* apply cold compresses to the nipple area.

BODY POSITION

Sleep on your back, with your upper body elevated, for at least the first week to ten days.

WALKING/EXERCISE

By the third day, you can probably start walking around the house. Many patients say that the third day is the most uncomfortable, so do not overdo it—listen to your body. If you feel tired, rest. Do not try to raise your arms. By the fourth day, you can possibly resume a light routine—no strenuous activity or lifting. Most physicians recommend that you wait a minimum of three to four weeks to resume aerobic exercise.

DRAINS

If drains were placed, these should be removed in two to three days. Removal of the drains may cause some discomfort, so consider taking your pain medication prior to this appointment.

INCISION LINES

You should receive instructions on the care of your incisions and when you can bathe. The sutures should be removed in seven to fourteen days. Your scars may remain red for four to six weeks and should gradually fade. Most scars become barely noticeable over time.

AGING AND GRAVITY

Remember—time marches on. The effects of aging and gravity will not stop after surgery. The more you wear a bra (optimally twenty-four hours a day), the less your breast tissue can stretch.

Pain

As with recovery times, pain tolerance is different for everyone. What one person may consider pain, another person may consider discomfort.

LEVEL OF PAIN/DISCOMFORT

Generally, with a breast reduction there is moderate discomfort during the postoperative period.

PAIN MEDICATION

Most discomfort can be controlled with pain medications you have been prescribed or Extra Strength Tylenol. You may find it necessary to take pain medication for the first three to four days.

Risks/Complications

Although problems are unlikely, you need to be aware of what can happen and what action you should take. Most risks/complications will be avoided if you

make an informed decision, choose a qualified physician, and follow your physician's instructions.

BLEEDING

Call your doctor immediately if there is any bleeding from the incisions.

INFECTION

Antibiotics are given to you intravenously during the procedure, and you will probably be instructed to take an oral antibiotic after surgery. Follow your doctor's instructions.

HEMATOMA

A hematoma, a collection of blood or fluid beneath the skin, is unlikely. However, if it does occur, it can be treated by drainage with a needle or with a compression garment.

ASYMMETRY

This problem may require another surgery.

CHANGES IN NIPPLE SENSATION

Nipple sensation may increase or decrease after a breast reduction. This change may or may not be permanent.

HYPERTROPHIC SCARRING

Report any signs immediately to your doctor; this scarring can be treated if caught early. (See "Definitions of Scarring/Skin Changes," page 56.)

HYPERPIGMENTED SCARRING

This scarring can be cosmetically tattooed. (See "Definitions of Scarring/Skin Changes," page 56.)

*B*row/Forehead Lift

A brow/forehead lift is specifically designed to help eliminate the lines that develop across the forehead and "frown" lines and to raise sagging eyebrows.

Different parts of the face age at different rates. Sagging eyebrows, forehead lines, and frown lines can make a person appear angry, sad, or tired. A brow/forehead lift can help rejuvenate a face and make it look more youthful. As with any cosmetic surgery procedure, it is extremely important to be informed. Since all options are not always presented, this section will help you be aware of the different techniques. Here are some interesting facts about the brow/forehead lift.

- If the brows are below the orbital rims, they are "ptotic" (drooping).

- A brow/forehead lift is often performed in conjunction with blepharoplasty (eyelid surgery), face-lift, and/or laser resurfacing.

Procedure

You must make some important decisions if you choose this procedure—the location of the incisions (technique), the position of the brows, and whether you want the corrugator muscles (between the brows) incised (cut) to eliminate the "scowl" lines. Educate yourself so that you can be a part of this decision-making process. The surgical options you choose may be determining factors in your physician selection. Remember that different doctors use different techniques and usually recommend the one(s) in which they are trained and experienced. In general, if you undergo a brow/forehead lift, here's what you can expect.

ANESTHESIA

A brow/forehead lift can be performed under local anesthesia with intravenous sedation or under general anesthesia. The type of anesthesia is dependent on the extent of the procedure to be performed, the doctor's choice, and the patient's medical history or desires.

TECHNIQUES

Three common methods are currently being used. The method your surgeon uses may be dependent on his training and experience.

Traditional or Bicoronal

This approach uses an incision behind the hairline—most often from ear to ear. The skin is separated from the underlying tissue and the corrugator muscles (between the brows) may be cut to eliminate the scowl lines. The skin and muscle are then lifted, and the excess (typically one-half to three-quarters of an inch) is trimmed. The incision is then closed with staples or sutures, which generally remain in place for eight to fourteen days. This method elevates the forehead hairline and can result in hair loss along the incision. If your hair is very fine or thin or you are balding, this may not be the technique you want to choose.

Endoscopic

This is a more advanced technique whereby an endoscope (a surgical camera on the end of a probe) and surgical tools are inserted into three to five small (two-centimeter) incisions made just behind the hairline. The periosteum (connective tissue covering the skull), muscle, and skin are separated from the bone; the corrugator muscles (between the brows) may be incised to eliminate the "scowl" lines; then the muscles and skin are lifted upward. The tissue is then "fixed" to the skull with sutures or screws, and the incisions are sutured or stapled. The forehead is not elongated with the endoscopic procedure, and the scars are very small. Hair loss along the incisions is uncommon.

Incisions for Males

In addition to the above techniques, a "direct" brow lift may be recommended for males. The incisions are made just above the eyebrows or in the forehead crease(s).

DRESSINGS

With any of these techniques, while you are still in the operating room, a "mummy wrap" dressing will likely be applied. This dressing may be removed by the doctor or nurse the next day during your first postoperative appointment.

STEPS IN THE BROW/FOREHEAD LIFT PROCEDURE

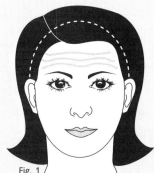

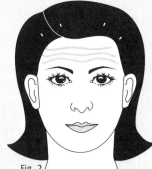

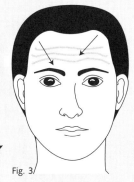

Fig. 1

Fig. 2

Fig. 3

Traditional or bicoronal: Incision behind (usually four finger widths) the hairline and most often from ear to ear (Figure 1). The skin is separated from the underlying tissue, the skin and muscle are lifted, and the excess is trimmed.

Endoscopic: A surgical camera on the end of a probe is inserted into three to five small incisions made just behind the hairline (Figure 2). The forehead skin, muscle, and tissue are separated from the bone, lifted upward, and then "fixed" to the skull with sutures or screws.

Direct: May be recommended for males. Incisions are placed just above the eyebrows or in the forehead creases (Figure 3).

LENGTH OF PROCEDURE

Any of these methods should take approximately two to two and one-half hours.

Prior to Surgery

Before surgery, you and your doctor will first make several important decisions. Then you will prepare for surgery and be given prescriptions and instructions. The following sections will give you an overview of the process.

ASSESSMENT

Your physician should evaluate and assess the sagging skin of your forehead in conjunction with the laxity and position of your eyebrows. In some cases, the upper lids might appear to be sagging when in actuality the problem is a sagging brow. A brow/forehead lift and eyelid lift (blepharoplasty) may be needed in combination to achieve the desired results. It is critical to have a

127

thorough assessment. Be absolutely clear and in agreement with your doctor about your desired look and the placement of your eyebrows.

PREOPERATIVE VISIT

You should be instructed to have certain lab tests, i.e., blood work, chest x-ray, EKG. (If you are also having a blepharoplasty, your physician may instruct you to have a thorough eye exam by an ophthalmologist.) For the lab tests, you may go to your family doctor, a hospital facility, or an independent lab. The physician you have chosen may arrange for the performance of these tests.

You may sign all of your surgical consent forms and be given pre- and postoperative instructions at this time. You should also be given your prescriptions for before and after surgery. Make sure that everything you and your physician have agreed on is stated on the consent form.

PRESCRIPTIONS

Some or all of these may be prescribed, in addition to others not listed:

- multivitamins—to be taken ten days to two weeks before and after surgery
- vitamin C—500 milligrams twice daily, to be taken ten days to two weeks before and after surgery
- pain medication
- antinausea medication
- oral antibiotics and/or ointment
- sleeping medication

Be sure to follow your doctor's instructions.

PRE- AND POSTOPERATIVE INSTRUCTIONS

These suggestions are intended to make you more comfortable and help you heal. To learn more, turn to the section on recovery in this chapter. Your doctor may have different or additional instructions. Follow them to the letter.

- Stop smoking, discontinue the use of alcohol, and stop taking vitamin E and any medications containing aspirin or ibuprofen (two weeks pre- and postoperative is usually recommended). Check with your doctor regarding any other medications (including homeopathic/herbal products) that you are currently taking.

- If you want to color your hair or have a permanent, do it a minimum of ten days prior to surgery. It will probably be about four to six weeks until you can color or have a permanent again.

- If you are having a bicoronal procedure and you wear your hair short, do not have it cut prior to the procedure. In that way, the longer hair will cover the incision until it heals.

- Be sure you understand how and when to take/apply your prescriptions.

- Know how to cleanse the surgical areas the night before or morning of your surgery.

- Do not have food (including gum or mints) or drink (including water) for a minimum of six to eight hours prior to surgery. (Follow your surgical facility's preoperative instructions.)

- Have someone drive you to and from surgery.

- Have someone stay with you the first night after surgery.

- Dressings, if the procedure requires them, should be applied by the doctor or nurse immediately after the procedure.

- Follow directions regarding any ointments to be applied.

- Do not sunbathe or use tanning beds at least two weeks prior to surgery. (For optimal skin care and health, these activities should be avoided completely.) After surgery, if you must be in the sun, take extra precautions to protect your forehead.

- Avoid aerobic activity for at least three weeks after surgery.

- Do not drive for at least forty-eight to seventy-two hours after surgery or while taking pain medication.

- Keep the head elevated at all times for at least the first week, optimally two weeks.

- Do not bend over for the first three weeks—if you must pick something up, squat with your knees bent.

- Lift nothing heavier than a small telephone book for at least two weeks.

- Expect some numbness in the forehead and scalp area for at least eight to twelve weeks. (The numbness should go away fairly quickly if your procedure was done endoscopically, more slowly if the coronal technique was performed.) Some patients have reported a level of numbness for up to a year or longer. However, the sensation tends to diminish over time.

- Be careful when using a hair dryer or curling iron because you cannot feel the heat.

- Your doctor may instruct you to apply cold compresses for twenty minutes every hour for a minimum of forty-eight hours.

- Rest and relax for the first week—your blood pressure must not be elevated.

- Do not apply makeup until your doctor instructs you.

Recovery

Everyone heals differently. Healing is affected by your genetics, your physical and emotional well-being, whether you smoke and/or drink alcohol, your pain tolerance, the extent of the surgery, and how well you follow the doctor's instructions. Plan on approximately seven to ten days for the initial healing period.

POSTOPERATIVE PHYSICIAN APPOINTMENTS

Your doctor may want to see you the day after surgery. That activity alone may be all you will want, or should do, that day. If a dressing was applied, this may be removed. Otherwise, do not remove this dressing unless you have been specifically instructed to do so by your physician. After your appointment, go home and rest. You may be given permission to shower that day or the next. Your appointments to return to the doctor's office should be in about one week to ten days (in two weeks for a bicoronal procedure) for suture/staple removal.

FIRST DAY POSTOPERATIVE

You may want to sleep the first day after surgery. For the first few hours after surgery, you may experience some nausea. You can expect your forehead and eyes to be swollen and mildly black and blue, and your forehead may appear very shiny. You may also have a headache or at least the feeling of wearing a very tight bathing cap. Expect some numbness in the forehead and scalp area for at least eight to twelve weeks.

SWELLING AND BRUISING

The swelling should lessen in the first few days, with some minor swelling remaining in the first weeks. You can also expect to be black and blue. This can last, on the average, anywhere from five days to several weeks but should diminish daily. Remember—everyone is different. You will probably notice that the swelling and bruising drop (travel lower in the face) over the first few days. Makeup will camouflage this, but check with your physician first.

NUMBNESS AND ITCHING

Expect some numbness in the forehead and scalp area for at least eight to twelve weeks. Some patients have reported a level of numbness for up to a year or longer. However, the sensation tends to diminish over time. Also, if the incision sites itch, gently rub the areas—do not scratch them. Ask your doctor if you can apply some cream or ointment to relieve the itching, and only use what is recommended.

COLD COMPRESSES

Cold compresses applied to the forehead/brow area may relieve some discomfort and can greatly reduce the swelling. These should be applied every hour for twenty minutes for a minimum of forty-eight hours (some doctors recommend seventy-two hours) after surgery. Ice should never be placed directly on the skin. Either use cold compresses or place a cloth between the ice bag and your skin. In some cases, your doctor may have instructed you *not* to use cold compresses. Follow your doctor's instructions.

BODY POSITION

It is important that you keep your head elevated at all times for at least the first seven days. Surround yourself with pillows or sleep on a recliner. Under no circumstances should you lie face down or bend over for the first three weeks. If you need to pick something up, squat with your knees bent. And do not pick up anything heavier than a small telephone book.

WALKING/EXERCISE

By the third day, you may be allowed to start walking around the house. Do not overdo it—listen to your body. If you feel tired, rest. By the fourth day, you can possibly resume some of your normal routine, except for strenuous activity or heavy lifting. Most physicians recommend that you wait a minimum of two to three weeks to resume aerobic exercise.

INCISION LINES

Your sutures/staples should be removed at your seven- to ten-day appointment (possibly in two weeks if you have had a bicoronal procedure). Your scars may remain red for four to six weeks and should gradually fade. Most scars tend to become barely noticeable over time. There may be temporary hair loss in the incision area(s), but this usually improves to some degree within four to six months.

Pain

As with recovery times, pain tolerance is different for everyone. What one person may consider pain, another person may consider discomfort.

LEVEL OF PAIN/DISCOMFORT

Generally, with a brow/forehead lift there is minimal discomfort during the postoperative period. Some people experience absolutely no discomfort at all.

PAIN MEDICATION

Most discomfort can be controlled with pain medications you have been prescribed or Extra Strength Tylenol. You may find it necessary to take pain medication for the first day or two only.

Risks/Complications

Although problems are unlikely, you need to be aware of what can happen and what action you should take. Most risks/complications will be avoided if you make an informed decision, choose a qualified physician, and follow your physician's instructions.

HEMATOMA

A hematoma, a collection of blood or fluid beneath the skin, is unlikely. However, if it does occur, it can be treated by drainage with a needle or with compression.

NERVE DAMAGE

Loss of sensation and/or movement is usually temporary.

RECURRENCE OF FOREHEAD LINES

Usually lines will not be as extensive or noticeable as before surgery if they come back.

HYPERTROPHIC SCARRING

Report any signs immediately to your doctor; this scarring can be treated if caught early. (See "Definitions of Scarring/Skin Changes," page 56.)

BROWS TOO HIGH

If you seem to have a surprised look, your brows may relax over time.

HAIR LOSS AT THE INCISIONS

This loss may or may not be permanent.

Cheek Augmentation—Malarplasty

Cheek augmentation is specifically designed to create more prominent cheekbones (malar bones), producing a more youthful appearance and/or achieving facial harmony.

The clinical term for cheek augmentation is malarplasty. In Western cultures, prominent cheekbones are considered aesthetically pleasing. This procedure is infrequently performed purely for cosmetic purposes because it can have a very dramatic effect on a patient's appearance. However, it may be necessary to bring the facial features into balance and harmony. Because of these issues, it is even more important for you to be totally informed. Here are some interesting facts about cheek augmentation.

- This procedure is often performed in conjunction with a rhinoplasty (nose reshaping), face-lift, liposuction of the chin and neck area, and/or chin augmentation/reduction.

- A number of synthetic materials are currently being used as cheek implants.

Procedure

You must make many important decisions if you choose this procedure—the location of the incisions, the type of material to be used, the size of the implants, and ultimately your desired look. Be as well informed as possible so that you can be a part of this decision-making process. The surgical options you choose may be determining factors in your physician selection. Remember that different doctors use different techniques and usually recommend the one(s) in which they are trained and experienced. In general, if you undergo a malarplasty, here's what you can expect.

IMPLANT MATERIALS

A number of synthetic materials are currently being used for cheek implants. They are made of materials that have been used for many years as prostheses. Some available products for implants include the following.

Silicone—solid or hollow silicone (tissue can grow into it). Silicone is manufactured in a wide range of consistencies from soft to hard.

Medpor—a textured, porous form of high-density polyethylene. The blood vessels grow into the implant, integrating it into the tissues.

Gore-Tex—pliable and microporous (tissue can grow into it).

ANESTHESIA

A malarplasty can be performed under local anesthesia with intravenous sedation or under general anesthesia. The type of anesthesia is dependent on the extent of the other procedure to be performed, the doctor's choice, and the patient's medical history or desires.

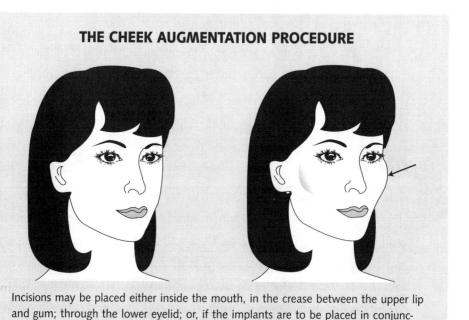

THE CHEEK AUGMENTATION PROCEDURE

Incisions may be placed either inside the mouth, in the crease between the upper lip and gum; through the lower eyelid; or, if the implants are to be placed in conjunction with a face-lift, they can be positioned through the face-lift incisions.

INCISIONS

There are three methods available for the placement of incisions:

- inside the mouth, in the crease between the upper lip and gum

- through the lower eyelid

- if the implants are to be placed in conjunction with a face-lift, through the face-lift incisions

Like anesthesia, the placement of the incisions is dependent on your doctor's training, experience, and preference, and your desires.

Whichever incision is used, pockets are created and the implants are placed in position under the tissue on the cheekbones. At that time, the implants may or may not be sutured or held in place with very small surgical screws. The incision is then sutured. If the incision is inside the mouth or inside the lower eyelid, absorbable sutures are used. If the incision is on the outside of the lower lid, the sutures may or may not be dissolvable.

DRESSINGS

While you are still in the operating room, the doctor or nurse may apply a tape dressing, which will have to remain in place for about five to seven days.

LENGTH OF PROCEDURE

This procedure should take approximately one and one-half to two hours.

Prior to Surgery

Before surgery, you and your doctor will first make several important decisions. Then you will prepare for surgery and be given prescriptions and instructions. The following sections will give you an overview of the process.

ASSESSMENT

Your physician should evaluate and assess the position of your cheekbones to determine facial harmony and balance. Your doctor may recommend cheek implants or a chin implant in combination with a face-lift to achieve the desired results. However, it is critical to have a thorough assessment. Be absolutely clear and in agreement with your doctor about your desired look. Cheek implants can produce a very dramatic change in your face, so it would be advisable to discuss with your doctor the actual size of the implant to be used. Discuss the implant material to be used as well.

PREOPERATIVE VISIT

You should be instructed to have certain lab tests, i.e., blood work, chest x-ray, EKG. You may go to your family doctor, a hospital facility, or an independent lab. The physician you have chosen may arrange for the performance of these tests.

You may sign all of your surgical consent forms and be given pre- and postoperative instructions at this time. You should also be given your prescriptions for before and after surgery. Make sure that everything you and your physician have agreed on, such as implant size, is stated on the consent form.

PRESCRIPTIONS

Some or all of these may be prescribed, in addition to others not listed:

- multivitamins—to be taken ten days to two weeks before and after surgery
- vitamin C—500 milligrams twice daily, to be taken ten days to two weeks before and after surgery
- pain medication
- antinausea medication
- oral antibiotics and/or ointment
- sleeping medication
- steroids (i.e., cortisone), to minimize swelling

  Be sure to follow your doctor's instructions.

PRE- AND POSTOPERATIVE INSTRUCTIONS

These suggestions are intended to make you more comfortable and help you heal. To learn more, turn to the section on recovery in this chapter. Your doctor may have different or additional instructions. Follow them to the letter.

- Stop smoking, discontinue the use of alcohol, and stop taking vitamin E and any medications containing aspirin or ibuprofen (two weeks pre- and postoperative is usually recommended). Check with your doctor regarding any other medications (including homeopathic/herbal products) that you are currently taking.

- Be sure you understand how and when to take/apply your prescriptions.
- Know how to cleanse the surgical areas the night before or morning of your surgery.
- Do not have food (including gum or mints) or drink (including water) for a minimum of six to eight hours prior to surgery. (Follow your surgical facility's preoperative instructions.)
- Have someone drive you to and from surgery.
- Have someone stay with you the first night after surgery (the first twenty-four hours, optimally).
- If dressings are required, they should be applied by the doctor or nurse immediately after the procedure. Do not get dressings wet.
- Follow directions regarding any ointments to be applied and/or cleansing of incisions. If incisions are inside the mouth, rinse your mouth as many times a day as directed.
- Do not sunbathe or use tanning beds at least two weeks prior to surgery. (For optimal skin care and health, these should be avoided completely.) After surgery, if you must be in the sun, take extra precautions to protect your face.
- Avoid aerobic activity for at least three weeks after surgery.
- Do not drive for at least twenty-four hours after surgery or while taking pain medication.
- Keep the head elevated at all times for at least the first week, optimally two weeks.
- For the first twenty-four hours, stay on a liquid diet and avoid food that is too hot.
- For about a week, avoid excessive talking, laughing, and heavy chewing (stay on a soft diet). Brush your teeth gently.
- Do not bend over for the first three weeks. If you must pick something up, squat with your knees bent.
- Lift nothing heavier than a small telephone book.
- Do not rub your cheeks—be gentle for a minimum of a month.

- Expect some numbness in the areas treated for eight to twelve weeks.

- Your doctor may instruct you to apply cold compresses for twenty minutes every hour for a minimum of forty-eight hours.

- Rest and relax for the first few days—your blood pressure must not be elevated.

- If your incisions are on the surface of the skin, they may itch as they start to heal. Do not scratch them.

- Avoid an accidental bump or injury to your cheek area for at least three weeks.

- Do not apply makeup until your doctor instructs you.

- Postpone any dental work until six months after cheek implant surgery.

Recovery

Everyone heals differently. Healing is affected by your genetics, your physical and emotional well-being, whether you smoke and/or drink alcohol, your pain tolerance, the extent of the surgery, and how well you follow the doctor's instructions. Plan on approximately one week to ten days for the initial healing period.

POSTOPERATIVE PHYSICIAN APPOINTMENTS

Your doctor may want to see you the day after surgery. That activity alone may be all you will want, or should do, that day. After your appointment, go home and rest. Your next appointment should be in five to seven days. If a dressing has been applied, this may be removed, and your stitches (if not absorbable) will likely be removed.

FIRST DAY POSTOPERATIVE

You may want to sleep the first day after surgery. You can expect your upper lip and cheek area to feel full, tight, and tender. The cheek area may be swollen and black and blue.

SWELLING AND BRUISING

The swelling should lessen daily, with some minor swelling remaining after the first few weeks. The bruising can last, on the average, anywhere from five days to several weeks but should diminish daily. Remember—everyone is different. You can apply makeup (regular and/or camouflage) after the sutures are removed or as instructed by your doctor.

NUMBNESS

Expect some numbness (as if your lip had been injected with Novocain) and a tight feeling in the treated areas for an average of eight to twelve weeks.

COLD COMPRESSES

Cold compresses applied to the face may relieve some of the discomfort and can greatly reduce the swelling. These should be applied every hour for twenty minutes for a minimum of forty-eight hours (some doctors recommend seventy-two hours) after surgery. Ice should never be placed directly on the skin. Either use cold compresses or place a cloth between the ice bag and your skin. In some cases, your doctor may have instructed you *not* to use cold compresses. Follow your doctor's instructions.

BODY POSITION

It is important that you keep your head elevated at all times for at least a week, optimally two. Surround yourself with pillows or sleep on a recliner if you must. Under no circumstances should you lie face down or bend over for the first three weeks. If you need to pick something up, squat with your knees bent; do not pick up anything heavier than a small telephone book. Avoid excessive talking, laughing, yawning, chewing, or other movements of the mouth for the first week. If you have mouth incisions, rinse your mouth as directed, and be very gentle when brushing your teeth. Do not touch your cheek area other than to wash very gently for the first three weeks.

WALKING/EXERCISE

By the third day, you may be allowed to start walking around the house. Do not overdo it—listen to your body. If you feel tired, rest. By the fourth day, you can possibly resume some of your normal routine, except for strenuous activity or heavy lifting. Most physicians recommend that you wait a minimum of two to three weeks to resume aerobic exercise.

INCISION LINES

If your incision is on the surface of the skin under the lower lid, the scars may remain red for four to six weeks and should gradually fade. Most scars become barely noticeable over time.

Pain

As with recovery times, pain tolerance is different for everyone. What one person may consider pain, another person may consider discomfort.

LEVEL OF PAIN/DISCOMFORT

Generally, with cheek implants there is minimal to moderate discomfort during the postoperative period. Some people experience absolutely no discomfort at all.

PAIN MEDICATION

Most discomfort can be controlled with pain medications you have been prescribed or Extra Strength Tylenol. You may find it necessary to take pain medication for the first day or two only.

Risks/Complications

Although problems are unlikely, you need to be aware of what can happen and what action you should take. Most risks/complications will be avoided if you make an informed decision, choose a qualified physician, and follow your physician's instructions.

INFECTION

Any fever, redness, severe constant pain, or uneven swelling should be reported immediately to your doctor.

IMPROPER POSITIONING OR SHIFTING OF IMPLANT

It is unlikely that the implant will shift. However, it is a simple procedure to reposition the implant.

NERVE DAMAGE

Loss of sensation and/or movement is usually temporary.

REJECTION OF IMPLANT

It is very unusual for an implant to be rejected by the body.

Chemical Peels

Peels work by chemically removing the top layer(s) of skin, resulting in an improvement of fine lines, wrinkles, skin tone, and irregular pigmentation that are unaffected by a face-lift.

The beauty industry is booming. That boom has attracted many newcomers to the business. As a result, procedures are being performed by individuals who may or may not have the proper training and experience. For this reason, it is even more important for you to be totally informed regarding chemical peels. Peels can range from mild peels or masks that can be done at home to medium peels that can be applied by a trained skin care specialist to the more radical treatments that only doctors should apply. The following section will help you sort through the differences. Here are some interesting facts about chemical peels.

- Peels can be applied to the whole face or a region of the face, such as around the eyes, or the area around the mouth (peri-orbital or peri-oral).

- Peels work best on the fine lines around the eyes and mouth.

- The fairer the skin, the less possibility of pigmentation problems.

- Peels should be avoided by anyone who scars easily or who has connective tissue disorders, such as lupus.

- A deep peel removes the top few layers of skin and shrinks the underlying collagen tissue, which results in a tightening of the skin.

- The skill and experience of the surgeon directly affect the results—complication rates are very low in the hands of a competent doctor.

- If you follow a healthy skin care program afterward, the improvements can last a lifetime.

Procedure

Numerous types of peels are available today. Many are marketed by physicians and skin care specialists by their brand names. However, all peels fall into one of four basic categories: over-the-counter, mild, medium, and deep peels. Your physician will guide you as to which peel will accomplish your desired goals. Many physicians nowadays are utilizing the erbium laser instead of medium chemical peels and the CO_2 laser as a replacement for deep chemical peels. (See "Laser Resurfacing," page 207.) However, there are many physicians and skin care specialists who still feel that chemical peels can be very effective. Chemical peels are also much less expensive than laser resurfacing. If you undergo a chemical peel, here's what you can expect.

TYPES OF CHEMICAL PEELS

The different types (strengths) of chemical peels are as follows. Which kind you choose will be determined by what you wish to accomplish.

Over-the-Counter Peels

These peels use alpha-hydroxy acids (AHAs), which are derived from apples, olives, or sugar cane. They loosen the dead cells from the surface of the skin (exfoliate) and speed up the skin's natural replenishing process. These can be applied daily at home. When applied, they give a slight burning or tingling sensation.

Glycolic Acid Peel

This is the mildest peel used by doctors or trained skin care specialists. It removes only the outer layers of the epidermis (outermost layer of skin). This peel will speed up the process of cell replacement, resulting in a slightly smoother and fresher look. Glycolic peels can be used on the face and neck. Often referred to as the "lunchtime" peel, these peels are administered once a week for two to six weeks. The strength of the acid and length of time it is left on the face are gradually increased. The acid is rinsed off thoroughly after being left on the face for two to five minutes. A soothing lotion is usually then applied.

The immediate sensation is that of a mild sunburn. Sensitive skin may swell and blister, or become irritated. If the patient experiences any burning sensation, it can be relieved by rinsing the skin periodically with cool water. Makeup must not be applied for several hours after the peel.

Trichloroacetic Peel (Trichloroacetic Acid/TCA)

This is a more aggressive peel used by doctors and should only be administered by the members of a doctor's staff who have had specific training. It removes the entire epidermis and only the most superficial portion of the dermis (the secondary layer of skin). It is usually done in sections and may cause discomfort. Different strengths may be used on different areas of your face. A very mild strength may be used on the neck.

The solution is applied with a cotton-tipped swab and left on the skin. Your skin initially turns white but quickly turns red (similar to a severe sunburn). The redness usually subsides in a few hours and will generally start to peel in three to five days.

You may be able to start to wear makeup again in about five days, although it usually takes one to two weeks for the skin to completely heal. Refrain from strenuous physical activity for about a week. The sun must be avoided for six to eight weeks afterward, and an increased sensitivity to the sun should be expected. The TCA peel takes approximately thirty minutes.

Phenol Peel (Carbolic Acid)

This is the most aggressive peel. It removes the entire epidermis, down to the middle of the dermis. It can be applied to the full face or a region of the face. Intravenous (IV) sedation or general anesthesia is usually necessary. Your vital signs must be monitored. The chemical is absorbed into the bloodstream so if it is applied too quickly, arrhythmias (irregular heartbeats) can occur. Therefore, the chemical is applied one section at a time, usually in fifteen-minute intervals.

With a cotton-tipped swab, the solution is applied and left on the face. A smaller amount is used around the eyes. Your face will initially turn white then bright red. A full-face phenol chemical peel takes approximately one and one-half hours.

Two techniques are used for protecting the face after a phenol peel. Some physicians apply a special dressing that stays on for a few days to a week; others apply an antiseptic ointment, which may be replaced in a few days with petroleum jelly.

Prior to Surgery

The following information pertains to a deep phenol chemical peel. Before the peel, you and your doctor will first make several important decisions. Then you will prepare for the peel and be given prescriptions and instructions. The following sections will give you an overview of the process.

ASSESSMENT

Your physician should discuss and assess your areas of concern, your skin's condition and type, and your history of healing. Patients who have experienced hyperpigmentation (a darkening of the skin) as a result of an injury or even pregnancy, an insect bite, or a pimple, may respond in the same way to a deep chemical peel. For these patients, most doctors prescribe skin lightening creams before and after the peel, inhibiting the formation of melanin (pigment).

AVOIDANCE OF SUN

The doctor should strongly warn patients to avoid the sun after the peel (even sunlight through a window must be strictly avoided). Pigment-producing cells are greatly reduced or changed so you are more susceptible to sunburn. After a deep chemical peel, getting a deep tan may be more difficult.

MEDICAL HISTORY DISCLOSURE

If you will be undergoing any type of facial peel, whether a chemical peel, dermabrasion, or laser resurfacing, it is imperative that you tell your doctor if you have a history of cold sores, shingles, or herpes infections, because these procedures can reactivate the virus. Many doctors routinely prescribe an oral antiviral medication. It is also extremely important to tell your doctor if you have taken any acne medication (such as Accutane) in the past year or if you have heart or kidney disease, diabetes, or any connective tissue disease, e.g., lupus, scleroderma.

PREOPERATIVE VISIT

You should be instructed to have certain lab tests, i.e., blood work, chest x-ray, EKG, urinalysis. You may go to your family doctor, a hospital facility, or an independent lab. The physician you have chosen may arrange for the performance of these tests.

146

You may sign all of your surgical consent forms and be given pre- and postoperative instructions at this time. You should also be given your prescriptions for before and after the peel. Make sure that everything you and your physician have agreed on is stated on your consent form.

PRESCRIPTIONS

Some or all of these may be prescribed, in addition to others not listed.

- antiviral medication—many physicians prescribe this whether or not you have a previous history of herpes infections
- Retin-A/alpha-hydroxy acids/topical vitamin solutions/topical steroids— some doctors pretreat their patients, because these products aid cell rejuvenation and exfoliation
- skin lightening creams—some doctors pretreat with these creams to prevent the possible temporary complication of skin darkening (transient hyperpigmentation)
- multivitamins—to be taken ten days to two weeks before and after surgery
- vitamin C—500 milligrams twice daily, to be taken ten days to two weeks before and after surgery
- pain medication
- antinausea medication
- oral antibiotics and/or ointment
- sleeping medication

    Be sure to follow your doctor's instructions.

PRE- AND POSTOPERATIVE INSTRUCTIONS

These suggestions are intended to make you more comfortable and help you heal. To learn more, turn to the section on recovery in this chapter. Your doctor may have different or additional instructions. Follow them to the letter.

- Stop smoking, discontinue the use of alcohol, and stop taking vitamin E and any medications containing aspirin or ibuprofen (two weeks before and after the phenol peel is usually recommended). Check with your doctor regarding any other medications (including homeopathic/herbal products) that you are currently taking.

- Be sure you understand how and when to take/apply your prescriptions.

- If general anesthesia or intravenous sedation is to be administered, do not have food (including gum or mints) or drink (including water) for a minimum of six to eight hours prior to a phenol peel. (Follow your surgical facility's preoperative instructions.)

- Have someone drive you to and from the trichloroacetic acid (TCA) peel or phenol peel.

- If the procedure requires dressings, these should be applied by the doctor or nurse immediately after the procedure.

- Keep the head elevated for about a week.

- Follow directions regarding any ointments/petroleum jelly to be applied.

- Do not sunbathe or use tanning beds at least two weeks prior to the peel. The doctor will also strongly warn you to avoid the sun after surgery (even sunlight through a window must be strictly avoided). Pigment-producing cells are greatly reduced or changed so you will be more susceptible to sunburn and getting a deep tan may be difficult.

- Avoid aerobic activity for ten days to two weeks after a phenol peel.

- Do not drive for at least twenty-four hours after a phenol peel and/or while taking pain medication.

Recovery

Everyone heals differently. Healing is affected by your genetics, your physical and emotional well-being, whether you smoke and/or drink alcohol, your pain tolerance, the extent of the peel, and how well you follow the doctor's instructions. For a phenol peel, plan on approximately eight to ten days before you will be able, or want, to go out in public (usually with some camouflage makeup for redness). The following recovery information pertains to a deep phenol chemical peel.

COMPLEX HEALING

Healing from a phenol chemical peel is complex with a demanding regimen of home care. It requires strict adherence to your doctor's pre- and postoperative instructions.

Your skin can be abnormally susceptible to infection for several weeks after the operation. Candida (yeast), herpes, and staphylococcus infections are particular dangers; all can cause skin changes that may result in a scar. Call your doctor instantly if you develop any signs of infection such as a high fever, severe localized pain, or swelling (after the initial swelling has subsided), or any kind of blistering or discharge, other than the clear oozing typical of the first few days.[1]

DRESSINGS/OINTMENT

Depending on the technique your doctor employs, your face should be coated either with an antibiotic ointment or petroleum jelly or with a thin dressing that maintains moisture (your face may be wrapped like a mummy). Your doctor may remove the dressing in a day or two.

FIRST DAY POSTOPERATIVE

After surgery, the areas that have been treated could be very sensitive and red and may start to swell immediately. Keep your head elevated at all times. Your eyes may be swollen almost shut and it may be uncomfortable to open your mouth. It is best to minimize the movement of your mouth in the first few weeks of healing. The swelling will usually start to go down in two to three days. Within about twenty-four hours, your skin will start to ooze a watery, yellowish serum. This will harden into a crust.

PHYSICIAN INSTRUCTIONS

There are a number of different techniques that physicians employ at this stage. *Follow your doctor's instructions to the letter.* Some doctors instruct the patient to wash the face a number of times during the day and then apply an ointment or petroleum jelly. Some doctors advise the application of cold compresses to dissolve the crusts; others instruct that you apply an ointment or petroleum jelly and/or apply cold compresses if a dressing has been applied on your face. If you are instructed to apply cold compresses, it is imperative that a barrier is between the compress and your skin—either a washcloth or the dressings. *Do not pick any crusts—this could cause scarring.*

---

[1] Tina Alster, M.D., and Lydia Preston, *Cosmetic Laser Surgery,* (Brooklyn: Alliance Publications, 1997).

Remember—do not apply anything to the treated areas except what is recommended or prescribed by your doctor. If you notice intense redness in one area and feel an underlying hardness or stiffness in that area, notify your doctor right away—you could be developing a hypertrophic (raised) scar. Unless treated early, a permanent scar can form.

FIRST WEEK TO TWO WEEKS POSTOPERATIVE

The oozing and crusting can require approximately one to two weeks to heal. Once new surface cells have built up (an average of eight days), the redness and sensitivity should lessen, and you can generally apply makeup. As your skin heals, it may feel tight and drier than normal, and begin to flake or appear chapped. You may also break out in bumps and pimples or may begin to itch. At three to four weeks, the treated areas may darken and turn brown (transient hyperpigmentation). All of these conditions can be treated, so notify your doctor immediately.

SWELLING AND REDNESS

The swelling should dissipate over the first few weeks. However, your skin could feel tight and dry for about six weeks. The redness should turn to pink, and it can then take (on average) up to three months for the pinkness to fade, maybe longer. Remember—everyone's healing time is different.

Pain

As with recovery times, pain tolerance is different for everyone. What one person may consider pain, another person may consider discomfort.

LEVEL OF PAIN/DISCOMFORT

Generally, with phenol peels the level of pain can be minimal to extreme (much of it is dependent on your adherence to the doctor's pre- and postoperative instructions).

PAIN MEDICATION

Most pain or discomfort can be controlled with pain medications you have been prescribed or Extra Strength Tylenol. You may find it necessary to take pain medication for the first day or two only. The dressing and/or ointment minimize, and in some cases eliminate, any discomfort.

Risks/Complications

Although problems are unlikely, you need to be aware of what can happen and what action you should take. Most risks/complications will be avoided if you make an informed decision, choose a qualified physician, and follow your physician's instructions.

SCARRING

Scarring could occur if the skin becomes infected or the peel goes too deep. It is of utmost importance to take/apply the antibiotics and/or antiviral drugs your doctor has prescribed.

DISCOLORATION

Blotchy patches (pigmentation changes) may appear, especially on darker complexions. This is temporary if treated with lightening creams as prescribed by your doctor.

ECTROPION OR SCLERAL SHOW

An ectropion is a condition in which the lower eyelid pulls away or rolls out. With scleral show, the lower lid droops enough so that the white of the eye below the cornea shows. These conditions can occur if the skin under the eyes tightens too much. Either condition may subside in three to six months as the skin relaxes. This condition most commonly occurs in patients who have had a transcutaneous (external incision) lower blepharoplasty (eyelid surgery).

CHANGE IN TEXTURE OF THE SKIN

The pores may be clogged. This problem usually clears up on its own or may need to be treated. Consult with your physician's skin care specialist.

VISION IMPAIRMENT OR BLINDNESS

If the acid is accidentally splashed into the eyes, your sight could be damaged. Ask your doctor how this complication is avoided.

ARRHYTHMIA (IRREGULAR HEARTBEATS)

This problem can occur if a phenol peel is applied too quickly; the patient must be monitored.

Chin Augmentation/Reduction

Chin augmentation/reduction is performed to bring the features of the face into balance and create facial harmony.

The clinical term for chin augmentation is "mentoplasty." It may be necessary to augment or reduce the chin in order to achieve facial harmony. A thorough evaluation is necessary because there a number of different techniques utilized for chin reductions and augmentations. Here are some interesting facts about chin augmentation/reduction.

- This procedure is often in conjunction with a rhinoplasty (nose reshaping), face-lift, liposuction in the chin and neck areas, and/or cheek augmentation.

- Reduction mentoplasty is an option if the chin is too large.

Procedure

You must make many important decisions if you choose this procedure—the technique to be used, the type of implant material, the size of the implant, and ultimately your desired look. The surgical options you choose may be determining factors in your physician selection. Educate yourself so that you can be a part of this decision-making process. Remember that different doctors use different techniques and usually recommend the one(s) in which they are trained and experienced. If you undergo a mentoplasty, here's what you can expect.

ANESTHESIA

A mentoplasty can be performed under local anesthesia with intravenous sedation or under general anesthesia. The type of anesthesia is dependent on the extent of other procedure(s) to be performed, the doctor's choice, and the patient's medical history or desires.

IMPLANT MATERIALS

A number of synthetic materials are currently being used for chin augmentations. They are made of materials that have been used for many years as prostheses. Some available products for implants include the following.

Silicone—solid or hollow silicone (tissue can grow into it). Manufactured in a wide range of consistencies from soft to hard.

Medpor—a textured, porous form of high-density polyethylene. The blood vessels grow into the implant, integrating it into the tissues.

Gore-Tex—pliable and microporous (tissue can grow into it). Very similar to the insulating material used inside the lining of ski jackets.

AUGMENTATION

A small incision is placed either (1) inside the mouth, in the crease between the lower lip and gum; or (2) in the crease under the chin. The placement of the incision is usually dependent on your doctor's training, experience, or preference. A pocket is created and the implant is placed in position under the tissue on the jawbone. At that time, the implant may or may not be sutured into place. If the incision is inside the mouth, absorbable sutures are used; if the incision is under the chin, absorbable sutures may or may not be used.

DRESSING

While you are still in the operating room, the doctor or nurse may apply a tape dressing, which may remain in place for about five to seven days.

LENGTH OF PROCEDURE

This procedure should take approximately one-half to one hour.

REDUCTION

This may be accomplished by trimming the bony tissue through an incision inside the mouth or under the chin. However, the lower jaw may need to be repositioned or set back or the upper jaw (maxilla) may need to be brought forward. It is only through a very thorough evaluation that the course of action is determined.

THE CHIN AUGMENTATION/REDUCTION PROCEDURE

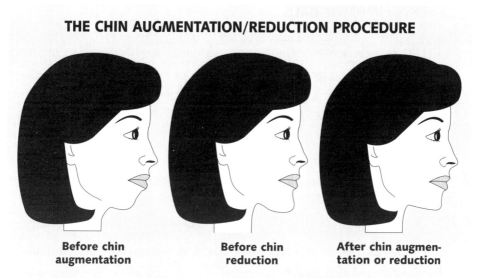

Before chin augmentation   **Before chin reduction**   **After chin augmentation or reduction**

For both procedures, a small incision is placed either (1) inside the mouth, in the crease between the lower lip and gum; or (2) in the crease under the chin. However, for chin reduction the lower jaw may need to be repositioned or set back, or the upper jaw (maxilla) may need to be brought forward.

Prior to Surgery

Before surgery, you and your doctor will first make several important decisions. Then you will prepare for surgery and be given prescriptions and instructions. The following sections will give you an overview of the process.

ASSESSMENT

Your physician should evaluate and assess the position of your chin to determine facial harmony and balance. Your doctor may recommend chin or cheek implants in combination with a face-lift and/or neck liposuction to achieve the desired results. Some patients who feel that they need a rhinoplasty (nose reshaping) may in fact only need a chin augmentation to achieve facial balance. It is critical to have a thorough assessment because a realignment of your jaw and/or teeth may be necessary. Be absolutely clear and in agreement with your doctor about your desired look. Discuss the material and the actual size of the implant to be used.

155

PREOPERATIVE VISIT

You should be instructed to have certain lab tests, i.e., blood work, chest x-ray, EKG. You may go to your family doctor, a hospital facility, or an independent lab. The physician you have chosen may arrange for the performance of these tests.

You may sign all of your surgical consent forms and be given pre- and postoperative instructions at this time. You should also be given your prescriptions for before and after surgery.

PRESCRIPTIONS

Some or all of these may be prescribed, in addition to others not listed.

- multivitamins—to be taken ten days to two weeks before and after surgery
- vitamin C—500 milligrams twice daily, to be taken ten days to two weeks before and after surgery
- pain medication
- antinausea medication
- oral antibiotics and/or ointment
- sleeping medication
- steroids (to minimize swelling)

Be sure to follow your doctor's instructions.

PRE- AND POSTOPERATIVE INSTRUCTIONS

These suggestions are intended to make you more comfortable and help you heal. To learn more, turn to the section on recovery in this chapter. Your doctor may have different or additional instructions. Follow them to the letter.

- Stop smoking, discontinue the use of alcohol, and stop taking vitamin E and any medications containing aspirin or ibuprofen (two weeks pre- and postoperative is usually recommended). Check with your doctor regarding any other medications (including homeopathic/herbal products) that you are currently taking.
- Be sure you understand how and when to take/apply your prescriptions.
- Know how to cleanse the surgical areas the night before or morning of your surgery.

- Do not have food (including gum or mints) or drink (including water) for a minimum of six to eight hours prior to surgery. (Follow your surgical facility's preoperative instructions.)

- Have someone drive you to and from surgery.

- Have someone stay with you the first night after surgery (the first twenty-four hours, optimally).

- Dressings, if these are required, should be applied by the doctor or nurse immediately after the procedure. Do not get dressings wet.

- Follow directions regarding any ointments to be applied and/or cleansing of incisions. If incisions are inside the mouth, rinse your mouth six times a day as directed.

- Do not sunbathe or use tanning beds at least two weeks prior to surgery. (For optimal skin care and health, these should be avoided completely.) If you must be in the sun, take extra precaution to protect your face.

- Avoid aerobic activity for at least three weeks after surgery.

- Do not drive for at least twenty-four hours after surgery and/or while taking pain medication.

- Keep the head elevated at all times for at least the first week, optimally two weeks.

- For the first twenty-four hours, stay on a liquid diet, and avoid food that is too hot.

- For about a week, avoid excessive talking, laughing, and heavy chewing (stay on a soft diet). Brush your teeth gently.

- Do not bend over for the first three weeks—if you must pick something up, squat with your knees bent.

- Lift nothing heavier than a small telephone book for one week.

- Do not rub your chin—be gentle for a minimum of a month.

- Expect some numbness in the areas treated for eight to twelve weeks.

- Your doctor may instruct you to apply cold compresses for twenty minutes every hour, for a minimum of forty-eight hours.

- Rest and relax for the first few days.

- If your incisions are on the surface of the skin, they may itch as they start to heal. Do not scratch them.

- Avoid injury to your chin area for about one month.

- Do not apply makeup until your doctor instructs you.

- Postpone any dental work for at least six weeks after placement of the implant.

Recovery

Everyone heals differently. Healing is affected by your genetics, your physical and emotional well-being, whether you smoke and/or drink alcohol, your pain tolerance, the extent of the surgery, and how well you follow the doctor's instructions. Plan on approximately one week to ten days for the initial healing period. However, if you have had jaw surgery, this can increase to six weeks.

POSTOPERATIVE PHYSICIAN APPOINTMENTS

Your doctor may want to see you the day after surgery. That activity alone may be all you will want, or should do, that day. After your appointment, go home and rest. Your next appointment should be in approximately five to seven days. Your stitches (if not absorbable) should be removed at that time.

FIRST DAY POSTOPERATIVE

You may want to sleep the first day after surgery. You can expect your lower lip and chin area to feel full, tight, and tender. The chin area may be swollen and black and blue.

SWELLING AND BRUISING

The swelling should lessen daily, with some minor swelling remaining after the first few weeks. The bruising can last, on the average, anywhere from five days to several weeks but should diminish daily. Remember—everyone is different. You can apply makeup (regular and/or camouflage) after the sutures are removed or as instructed by your doctor.

NUMBNESS

Expect some numbness (as if your lip had been injected with Novocain) and a tight feeling in the treated areas for an average of eight to twelve weeks.

COLD COMPRESSES

Cold compresses applied to the face may relieve some of the discomfort and can greatly reduce the swelling. These should be applied every hour for twenty minutes for a minimum of forty-eight hours (some doctors recommend seventy-two hours) after surgery. Ice should never be placed directly on the skin. Either use cold compresses or place a cloth between the ice bag and your skin. In some cases, your doctor may have instructed you *not* to use cold compresses. Follow your doctor's instructions.

BODY POSITION

It is important that you keep your head elevated at all times for at least the first week. Surround yourself with pillows or sleep on a recliner if you must. Under no circumstances can you lie face down for the first three weeks. If you need to pick something up, squat with your knees bent and do not pick up anything heavier than a small telephone book. Avoid excessive talking, laughing, or chewing for the first week. If you have mouth incisions, rinse your mouth as directed, and be very gentle when brushing your teeth. For the first three weeks, do not touch your chin other than to wash very gently.

WALKING/EXERCISE

By the third day, you may be allowed to start walking around the house. Do not overdo it—listen to your body. If you feel tired, rest. By the fourth day, you can possibly resume some of your normal routine, except for strenuous activity or heavy lifting. Most physicians recommend that you wait a minimum of two to three weeks to resume aerobic exercise.

DRESSINGS

If you have dressings and/or tape, you may be instructed not to get them wet.

INCISION LINES

If your incision is under the chin, the scar may remain red for four to six weeks and should gradually fade. Most scars become barely noticeable over time.

Pain

As with recovery times, pain and/or discomfort tolerance is different for everyone. What one person may consider pain, another person may consider discomfort.

LEVEL OF PAIN/DISCOMFORT

Generally, with a chin implant there is minimal to moderate discomfort during the postoperative period. Some people experience absolutely no discomfort at all.

PAIN MEDICATION

Most discomfort can be controlled with pain medications you have been prescribed or Extra Strength Tylenol. You may find it necessary to take pain medication for the first day or two only.

Risks/Complications

Although problems are unlikely, you need to be aware of what can happen and what action you should take. Most risks/complications will be avoided if you make an informed decision, choose a qualified physician, and follow your physician's instructions.

INFECTION

Any fever, redness, severe constant pain, or uneven swelling should be reported immediately to your doctor.

IMPROPER POSITIONING OR SHIFTING OF IMPLANT

It is unlikely that the implant will shift. However, if it does occur, it is a simple procedure to reposition.

NERVE DAMAGE

Loss of sensation and/or movement of the lip and/or chin is usually temporary.

REJECTION OF IMPLANT

It is very unusual for an implant to be rejected by the body.

$\mathcal{D}$ermabrasion

Dermabrasion works by mechanically removing the entire epidermis and varying depths of the dermis. It smoothes out wrinkles, acne, and raised scars on the face.

Dermabrasion is a surgical procedure used to treat uneven areas of the face; for example, acne scarring. The whole face or a region of the face, such as the area around the eyes or the mouth, can be treated. However, it is usually used for small areas of the face. With any surgical procedure, it is important to be informed. However, because of the possibility of scarring, it is even more important to educate yourself. The following section will help you. Here are some interesting facts about dermabrasion.

- A hand-held, motorized device called a "dermabrader" (much like a rotating sander) is used.
- The fairer the skin, the less possibility of pigmentation problems.
- Dermabrasion can be combined with a chemical peel in a procedure known as "chemabrasion" to remove deep wrinkles.
- Dermabrasion costs less than laser resurfacing.

Procedure

Even though the use of dermabrasion has diminished as more and more physicians are utilizing lasers, many physicians still feel that it can be an effective tool in certain cases. Some physicians may use it in conjunction with the laser and other procedures, such as dermal grafting. The results of dermabrasion are directly affected by the skill and experience of your physician, as there is a significant risk of scarring, especially with aggressive dermabrasion. However, if you undergo dermabrasion, here's what you can expect.

ANESTHESIA

Depending on the extent of the procedure, the areas may be numbed with a freezing spray or other topical or local anesthetic. The doctor then literally sands away the top layer(s) of skin with a dermabrader.

DRESSING

Two techniques are used for protecting the face after dermabrasion. Some physicians apply a special dressing that stays on for a few days to a week; others apply an antiseptic ointment, which may be replaced in a few days with petroleum jelly.

Prior to Surgery

Before dermabrasion, you and your doctor will first make several important decisions. Then you will prepare for surgery and be given prescriptions and instructions. The following sections will give you an overview of the process.

ASSESSMENT

Your physician should discuss and assess your areas of concern, your skin's condition and type, and your history of healing. Patients who have experienced hyperpigmentation (a darkening of the skin) as a result of pregnancy or an injury (even an insect bite or pimple), could respond in the same way to dermabrasion. For these patients, most doctors prescribe skin lightening creams that inhibit the formation of melanin pigment before and after the dermabrasion.

EXPOSURE TO SUN

The doctor should also strongly warn patients to avoid the sun after surgery (even sunlight through a window must be strictly avoided). Pigment-producing cells are greatly reduced or changed, making you more susceptible to sunburn. After dermabrasion, getting a deep tan is very difficult.

MEDICAL HISTORY DISCLOSURE

If you will be undergoing any type of facial peel, whether dermabrasion, a chemical peel, or laser resurfacing, it is imperative that you tell your doctor if you have a history of cold sores, shingles, or herpes infections, because these procedures can reactivate the virus. Many doctors routinely prescribe an oral antiviral medication. It is also extremely important to tell your doctor if you have taken any acne medication (such as Accutane) in the past year or if you have heart or kidney disease, diabetes, or any connective tissue disease, e.g., lupus, scleroderma.

PREOPERATIVE VISIT

You should be instructed to have certain lab tests, i.e., blood work, chest x-ray, EKG. You may go to your family doctor, a hospital facility, or an independent lab. The physician you have chosen may arrange for the performance of these tests.

You may sign all of your surgical consent forms, and be given pre- and post-operative instructions at this time. You should also be given your prescriptions for before and after surgery. Make sure that everything you and your physician have agreed on is stated on your consent form.

PRESCRIPTIONS

Some or all of these may be prescribed, in addition to others not listed.

- antiviral medication—many physicians prescribe this, whether or not you have a previous history of herpes infections
- Retin-A/alpha-hydroxy acids/topical vitamin solutions/topical steroids—some doctors pretreat their patients because these products aid cell rejuvenation and exfoliation
- skin lightening creams—some doctors pretreat with these creams to prevent the possible temporary complication of skin darkening (transient hyperpigmentation)
- multivitamins—to be taken ten days to two weeks before and after surgery
- vitamin C—500 milligrams twice daily, to be taken ten days to two weeks before and after surgery
- pain medication
- antinausea medication
- oral antibiotics and/or ointment
- sleeping medication

Be sure to follow your doctor's instructions.

163

PRE- AND POSTOPERATIVE INSTRUCTIONS

These suggestions are intended to make you more comfortable and help you heal. To learn more, turn to the section on recovery in this chapter. Your doctor may have different or additional instructions. Follow them to the letter.

- Stop smoking, discontinue the use of alcohol, and stop taking vitamin E and any medications containing aspirin or ibuprofen (two weeks before and after the dermabrasion is usually recommended). Check with your doctor regarding any other medications (including homeopathic/herbal products) that you are currently taking.

- Be sure you understand how and when to take/apply your prescriptions.

- If general anesthesia or intravenous sedation is to be administered, do not have food (including gum or mints) or drink (including water) for a minimum of six to eight hours prior to dermabrasion. (Follow your surgical facility's preoperative instructions.)

- Have someone drive you to and from the dermabrasion.

- Dressings, if the procedure requires them, should be applied by the doctor or nurse immediately after the procedure.

- Keep the head elevated.

- Follow directions regarding any ointments/petroleum jelly to be applied.

- Do not sunbathe or use tanning beds at least two weeks prior to the procedure. The doctor should also strongly warn patients to avoid the sun after surgery (even sunlight through a window must be strictly avoided). Pigment-producing cells are greatly reduced or changed, making you more susceptible to sunburn.

- Avoid aerobic activity for ten days to two weeks after dermabrasion.

- Do not drive for at least twenty-four hours after dermabrasion and/or while taking pain medication.

Recovery

Everyone heals differently. Healing is affected by your genetics, your physical and emotional well-being, whether you smoke and/or drink alcohol, your pain tolerance, the extent of the surgery, and how well you follow the doctor's instructions. Plan on approximately one to two weeks before you will be able, or want, to go out in public (usually with some camouflage makeup for redness).

COMPLEX HEALING

Healing from dermabrasion is complex, with a demanding regimen of home care. It requires strict adherence to your doctor's pre- and postoperative instructions.

> *Your skin can be abnormally susceptible to infection for several weeks after the operation. Candida (yeast), herpes, and staphylococcus infections are particular dangers; all can cause skin changes that may result in a scar. Call your doctor instantly if you develop any signs of infection such as a high fever, severe localized pain, or swelling (after the initial swelling has subsided), or any kind of blistering or discharge, other than the clear oozing typical of the first few days.*[1]

DRESSINGS/OINTMENT

Depending on the technique your doctor employs, your face could be coated either with an antibiotic ointment or petroleum jelly or with a thin dressing that maintains moisture (your face may be wrapped like a mummy). Your doctor may remove the dressing in a day or two.

FIRST DAY POSTOPERATIVE

After surgery, the areas that have been treated could be very sensitive and red and may start to swell immediately. Keep your head elevated at all times. It is best to minimize the movement of your mouth in the first few weeks of healing. The swelling usually starts to go down in two to three days. Within twenty-four hours, your skin will start to ooze a watery, yellowish serum. This will harden into a crust.

PHYSICIAN INSTRUCTIONS

There are a number of different techniques that doctors employ at this stage. *Follow your doctor's instructions to the letter.* Some doctors instruct the patient to wash the face a number of times during the day and then apply an ointment

---

[1] Tina Alster, M.D., and Lydia Preston, *Cosmetic Laser Surgery*, (Brooklyn: Alliance Publications, 1997).

or petroleum jelly; some doctors advise the application of cold compresses to dissolve the crusts; others instruct that you apply an ointment or petroleum jelly and/or apply cold compresses if a dressing has been applied on your face. If you are instructed to apply cold compresses, it is imperative that something is between the compress and your skin—either a washcloth or the dressings. *Do not pick any crusts—this could cause scarring.*

Remember—do not apply anything to the treated areas except what is recommended or prescribed by your doctor. If you notice intense redness in one area and feel an underlying hardness or stiffness in that area, notify your doctor immediately—you could be developing a hypertrophic (raised) scar. Unless treated early, a permanent scar can form.

FIRST WEEK TO TWO WEEKS POSTOPERATIVE

The oozing and crusting can require approximately one to two weeks to heal. Once new surface skin cells have built up (an average of eight days), the redness and sensitivity should lessen, and you can generally apply makeup. As your skin heals, it may feel tight and drier than normal and begin to flake or appear chapped. You may also break out in bumps and pimples due to clogged pores or may begin to itch. At three to four weeks, the treated areas may darken and turn brown (transient hyperpigmentation). All of these conditions can be treated, so notify your doctor immediately.

SWELLING AND REDNESS

The swelling should dissipate over the first few weeks. However, your skin could feel tight and dry for about six weeks. The redness should turn to pink, and it can then take (an average) up to three months for the pinkness to fade, maybe longer. Remember—everyone's healing time is different.

Pain

As with recovery times, pain tolerance is different for everyone. What one person may consider pain, another person may consider discomfort.

LEVEL OF PAIN/DISCOMFORT

Generally, with dermabrasion, the level of pain can be moderate to extreme (much of it is dependent on your adherence to the doctor's pre- and postoperative instructions).

PAIN MEDICATION

Most pain or discomfort can be controlled with pain medications you have been prescribed or Extra Strength Tylenol. You may find it necessary to take pain medication for the first day or two only. The dressing and/or ointment minimize, and in some cases eliminate, any discomfort.

Risks/Complications

Although problems are unlikely, you need to be aware of what can happen and what action you should take. Most risks/complications will be avoided if you make an informed decision, choose a qualified physician, and follow your physician's instructions.

SCARRING

A greater potential for scarring exists in areas that have been aggressively treated. Scarring can also can occur if the skin becomes infected. It is of utmost importance to take/apply the antibiotics and/or antiviral drugs your doctor has prescribed.

DISCOLORATION

Blotchy patches (pigmentation changes) may appear, especially on darker complexions. This is temporary if treated with lightening creams as prescribed by your doctor.

CHANGE IN TEXTURE OF SKIN

The pores may be clogged. This problem usually clears up on its own or may need to be treated. Consult with your physician's skin care specialist.

$\mathcal{E}$*ar Pinning–Otoplasty*

Otoplasty is specifically designed to "pin back" or reposition protruding ears and create natural-looking folds and convolutions.

Otoplasty is very rewarding because of the visual improvement and psychological satisfaction. It is one of the few cosmetic surgery procedures performed on children; they can be as young as kindergarten age. This procedure also has great appeal for men, because most wear their hair short. As with any surgical procedure, it is extremely important to be informed. The following section will help you. Here are some interesting facts about otoplasty.

- Sometimes only one ear protrudes. However, surgery may need to be performed on both ears to attain maximum results if any change to the convolutions and/or folds is necessary.

- Perfect symmetry is rarely achieved.

Procedure

Patients choose otoplasty because they have felt self-conscious about their ears all of their lives. Many parents choose otoplasty for their young children. It is usually performed before the children start school in order to avoid the psychological problems they may incur as a result of other children's teasing. Remember that different doctors use different techniques. If you undergo an otoplasty, here's what you can expect.

ANESTHESIA
An otoplasty can be performed under local anesthesia with intravenous sedation or under general anesthesia. The type of anesthesia is dependent on the extent of the procedure to be performed, the age of the patient, the doctor's choice, and the patient's desires or medical history.

INCISIONS

Incisions (two to three inches long) are made in the natural creases behind the ears. The cartilage of the ear is weakened and bent into its new shape. Cartilage may or may not be removed. Permanent sutures are then placed in the cartilage to hold it in its new position and bring the ear closer to the head.

DRAINS AND DRESSINGS

Drains may or may not be inserted. While you are still in the operating room, the doctor or nurse will probably wrap your head in a turban-type of dressing that covers your ears. This may be removed the next day.

LENGTH OF PROCEDURE

This procedure takes approximately one to two hours. Children may be required to stay in the surgical facility for twenty-four hours to be monitored.

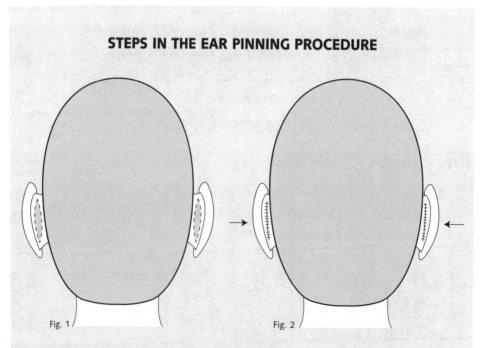

STEPS IN THE EAR PINNING PROCEDURE

Fig. 1

Fig. 2

Incisions (two to three inches) are made in the natural creases behind the ears. Cartilage may or may not be removed (Figure 1). Permanent sutures are then placed in the cartilage to hold it in its new position and bring the ear closer to the head (Figure 2).

Prior to Surgery

Before surgery, you and your doctor will first make several important decisions. Then you will prepare for surgery and be given prescriptions and instructions. The following sections will give you an overview of the process.

ASSESSMENT

Your physician evaluates and assesses the folds and convolutions of your ears in conjunction with their position. Be absolutely clear and in agreement with your doctor about your desired look.

PREOPERATIVE VISIT

You should be instructed to have certain lab tests, i.e., blood work, chest x-ray, EKG. You may go to your family doctor, a hospital facility, or an independent lab. The physician you have chosen may arrange for the performance of these tests.

You may sign all of your surgical consent forms and be given pre- and postoperative instructions at this time. You should also be given your prescriptions for before and after surgery. Make sure that everything that you and your physician have agreed on is stated on your consent form.

PRESCRIPTIONS

Some or all of these may be prescribed, in addition to others not listed.

- multivitamins—to be taken ten days to two weeks before and after surgery
- vitamin C—500 milligrams twice daily, to be taken ten days to two weeks before and after surgery
- pain medication
- antinausea medication
- oral antibiotics and/or ointment

Be sure to follow your doctor's instructions.

PRE- AND POSTOPERATIVE INSTRUCTIONS

These suggestions are intended to make you more comfortable and help you heal. To learn more, turn to the section on recovery in this chapter. Your doctor may have different or additional instructions. Follow them to the letter.

- Stop smoking, discontinue the use of alcohol, and stop taking vitamin E and any medications containing aspirin or ibuprofen (two weeks pre- and post-operative is usually recommended). Check with your doctor regarding any other medications (including homeopathic/herbal products) that you are currently taking.

- If you want to color your hair or have a permanent, have it done a minimum of ten days prior to surgery. It could be about four to six weeks until you can color or have a permanent again.

- Be sure you understand how and when to take/apply your prescriptions.

- Know how to cleanse the surgical areas the night before or morning of your surgery.

- Do not have any food (including gum or mints) or drink (including water) for a minimum of six to eight hours prior to surgery. (Follow your surgical facility's preoperative instructions.)

- Have someone drive you to and from surgery.

- Have someone stay with you the first night after surgery (the first twenty-four hours, optimally).

- Avoid straining during a bowel movement.

- Dressings, if the procedure requires them, should be applied by the doctor or nurse immediately after the procedure.

- Follow directions regarding any ointments to be applied and/or cleansing of incisions.

- Avoid aerobic activity for at least one week after surgery.

- Avoid contact sports for six weeks.

- Do not drive for at least twenty-four hours after surgery and/or while taking pain medication.

- Keep the head elevated at all times for at least the first week, optimally two weeks.

- Do not bend over for the first three weeks—if you must pick something up, squat with your knees bent.

- Lift nothing heavier than a small telephone book.

- Expect some numbness in and around your ears. Be careful when using a hair dryer or curling iron because you cannot feel the heat.

- Eyeglasses should not be worn for a week or two after surgery.

- Your doctor may instruct you to apply cold compresses for twenty minutes every hour for a minimum of forty-eight hours.

- Rest and relax for the first week.

Recovery

Everyone heals differently. Healing is affected by your genetics, your physical and emotional well-being, whether you smoke and/or drink alcohol, your pain tolerance, the extent of the surgery, and how well you follow the doctor's instructions. Plan on approximately five to ten days for the initial healing period.

POSTOPERATIVE PHYSICIAN APPOINTMENTS

Your doctor may want to see you the day after surgery. That activity alone could be all you will want, or should do, that day. If a dressing was applied, this may be removed. You may at this time be instructed to wear a protective covering, stocking cap, or headband pulled down over your ears while sleeping for another two weeks or longer. After your appointment, go home and rest. You may be given permission to shower that day or the next. However, if your dressing has not been removed, do not get it wet. You should have an appointment to return to the doctor's office in about one week to ten days.

FIRST DAY POSTOPERATIVE

You may want to sleep the first day after surgery. For the first few hours after surgery, you may experience some nausea. Expect some numbness in the area around your ears. As with all surgery, there could be some swelling and bruising.

SWELLING AND BRUISING

The swelling should lessen in the first few days with some minor swelling remaining in the first weeks. You can also expect to be black and blue. This can last, on the average, anywhere from five days to several weeks but will diminish daily. Remember—everyone is different. You may notice that the swelling and bruising drop (travel lower in the face) over the first few days. This is normal.

DRESSINGS

If a dressing was applied, this may be removed the day after surgery at your physician's office. You may at this time be instructed to wear a protective covering, stocking cap, or headband pulled down over your ears while sleeping for another two weeks or longer. When the dressings are first removed, it may appear that your ears are too close to your head. In time this dissipates and your ears will return to the new normal position.

COLD COMPRESSES

Cold compresses applied to the ear area may relieve some of the discomfort and can greatly reduce the swelling. These should be applied every hour for twenty minutes for a minimum of forty-eight hours (some doctors recommend seventy-two hours) after surgery. Ice should never be placed directly on the skin. Either use cold compresses or place a cloth between the ice bag and your skin. In some cases, your doctor may have instructed you *not* to use cold compresses. Follow your doctor's instructions.

BODY POSITION

It is imperative that you keep your head elevated at all times for at least the first week, optimally two weeks. Surround yourself with pillows or sleep on a recliner if you must. Try to avoid any type of pressure on the ear area. Under no circumstances should you lie face down, or bend over for the first three weeks. If you need to pick something up, squat with your knees bent. And do not pick up anything heavier than a small telephone book.

WALKING/EXERCISE

By the third day, you may be allowed to start walking around the house. Do not overdo it—listen to your body. If you feel tired, rest. By the fourth day, you can possibly resume some of your normal routine, except for strenuous activity or heavy lifting. Most physicians recommend that you wait a minimum of two to three weeks to resume aerobic exercise. However, no matter what the activity, the ears must be protected against injury for at least six weeks.

INCISION LINES

During the first few weeks, you may be instructed to cleanse the incision area with hydrogen peroxide applied with a cotton-tipped swab. Most of the sutures used behind the ears to close the incision usually dissolve. If they are nondissolvable, they are generally removed in about one to two weeks. The sutures placed in the cartilage to create the new shape are permanent and therefore not removed. However, do not bend the ear. Your scars may remain red for four to six weeks and should gradually fade. Most scars become barely noticeable over time, especially since they are hidden behind the ear.

Pain

As with recovery times, pain tolerance is different for everyone. What one person may consider pain, another person may consider discomfort.

LEVEL OF PAIN/DISCOMFORT

Generally, with otoplasty there is minimal to moderate discomfort during the postoperative period. However, be aware that your ears come in contact with many objects as you go about your day—combing your hair, dressing, hugging, and sleeping. Patients are cautioned that any bump can be quite uncomfortable.

PAIN MEDICATION

Most discomfort can be controlled with pain medications you have been prescribed or Extra Strength Tylenol. You may find it necessary to take pain medication for the first day or two only.

Risks/Complications

Although problems are unlikely, you need to be aware of what can happen and what action you should take. Most risks/complications will be avoided if you make an informed decision, choose a qualified physician, and follow your physician's instructions.

NERVE DAMAGE

Loss of sensation is usually temporary.

INFECTION
Infection is unlikely if your doctor's instructions are followed.

HYPERTROPHIC SCARRING
This type of scarring is rare. (See "Definitions of Scarring/Skin Changes," page 56.)

REACTION TO THE STITCHES
Contact your physician immediately. Medication may be prescribed.

ASYMMETRY
Perfection is rarely achieved.

*E*yelids–Blepharoplasty

Blepharoplasty is the term for the procedure that corrects aging of the eyelids. Excess skin and fat pads are removed from upper and/or lower eyelids.

Different parts of the face age at different rates. Droopy, sagging eyelids and bulging fat pads, which can be the result of gravity and/or heredity, can make a person appear sad and tired. Since the eyes are such a prominent facial feature, a blepharoplasty can help rejuvenate the face and make it look more youthful and refreshed. As with any cosmetic surgery procedure, it is extremely important to be informed. Since the media does not always present all the options that are available, this section will help you be aware of the different techniques. Here are some important facts about blepharoplasty.

- It is the second most common procedure performed on both men and women.

- Upper and lower "blephs" can be performed in conjunction with each other, or by themselves.

- Eyelid surgery cannot eliminate the wrinkles known as "crow's feet." Laser resurfacing or a chemical peel would be necessary.

- The position of the brows is not changed with eyelid surgery alone.

- This procedure is performed quite often in conjunction with other facial procedures, such as a brow/forehead lift, face-lift, or laser resurfacing.

- People of all ages seek this procedure.

Procedure

You must make some important decisions if you choose this procedure—the location of the incisions (technique) and your desired look. Educate yourself so that you can be a part of this decision-making process. The surgical options you choose may be determining factors in your physician selection. Remember that different doctors use different techniques and usually recommend the one(s) in which they are trained and experienced. In general, if you undergo a blepharoplasty, here's what you can expect.

ANESTHESIA

Blepharoplasty can be performed under local anesthesia with intravenous sedation or general anesthesia. The type of anesthesia is dependent on the extent of the procedure to be performed, the doctor's choice, and the patient's medical history or desires.

UPPER LID TECHNIQUE

Your doctor may make marks on your lids while you are in a sitting position. You may also be given special eye drops that numb the eyes and/or antiseptic eye drops to help prevent infection. If a laser is being used to make the incisions, your eyes may be shielded with steel eye covers. An incision is made (with a scalpel or laser) in the normal crease of your eyelid and the excess skin is removed. This exposes the underlying muscle and fat pads. A small amount of muscle is removed so that the eyelid crease is defined. The incision is then stitched closed. After surgery, some doctors apply small strips of tape to the eyelids; some do not. If used, these tapes will remain in place for three to seven days and will be removed by your doctor.

LOWER LID TECHNIQUES

There are two methods currently being used. The method your surgeon uses may be dependent on his/her training, experience, and/or preference. It is suggested that you inquire as to the reasons why the traditional versus the transconjunctival technique would be used in your particular case.

Traditional or Transcutaneous

This may be the approach with which your surgeon is most familiar and/or experienced. Today, it may also be used if there is a large amount of excess skin below the eyes. An incision is made just below the lower lashes, the fat pads are exposed and removed, and any excess skin and muscle are removed. This method, using the external incision, carries an increased potential for a complication known

STEPS IN THE EYELIDS PROCEDURE

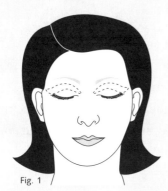

Fig. 1

Upper Lids: The incision is made in the normal crease of the eyelid (Figure 1). The fat pads are removed, as well as a small amount of muscle.

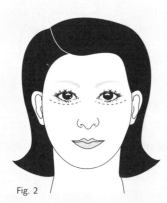

Fig. 2

Lower Lids: *Traditional (External)*—The incision is made just below the lower lashes (Figure 2). The fat pads, along with any excess skin and muscle, are removed.

Transconjunctival—The incision is made inside the lower lid (Figure 3). The fat pads are removed. If there is excess skin, a small pinch can be removed and stitched with very fine sutures. Otherwise, there are no sutures.

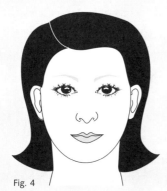

Fig. 3

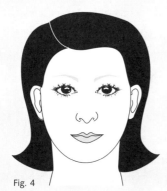

Fig. 4

Postoperatively, the upper lids are not sagging, and the area under the eyes is no longer puffy in appearance (Figure 4).

179

as ectropion, whereby the lower lid pulls down so far that the whites of the eyes show. Sometimes a complication such as ectropion can correct itself over time (usually within three to six months) or it may be permanent.

Transconjunctival

This method is achieved with an incision on the inside of the lower lid. The fat pads are exposed and excess fat is removed. If there is excess skin, a small pinch (from the outside) can be removed and stitched with very fine sutures. This approach is gaining more popularity today. There is less risk of ectropion, since the muscle is generally not disturbed, and a significant amount of skin is not removed.

LENGTH OF PROCEDURE

Upper lid blepharoplasty should take approximately one hour. Lower lid blepharoplasty (either traditional or transconjunctival) should take approximately one hour.

Prior to Surgery

Before surgery, you and your doctor will first make several important decisions. Then you will prepare for surgery and be given prescriptions and instructions. The following sections will give you an overview of the process.

ASSESSMENT

Your physician should evaluate and assess the sagging skin of your lids in conjunction with the laxity and position of your eyebrows. In some cases, the upper lids might appear to be sagging, when in actuality the problem is a sagging brow. An eyelid lift and a forehead/brow lift may be needed in combination to achieve the desired results. It is critical to have a thorough assessment.

PREOPERATIVE VISIT

You should be instructed to have a thorough eye exam by an ophthalmologist and certain lab tests, i.e., blood work, chest x-ray, EKG. If you do not have an ophthalmologist, your doctor should refer you to one. For the lab tests, you may go to your family doctor, an independent lab, or hospital facility. The physician you have chosen may arrange for the performance of these tests.

You may sign all of your surgical consent forms and be given pre- and post-operative instructions at this time. You should also be given your prescriptions for before and after surgery. Make sure that everything you and your physician have agreed on is stated on your consent form.

PRESCRIPTIONS

Some or all of these may be prescribed, in addition to others not listed.

- multivitamins—to be taken ten days to two weeks before and after surgery
- vitamin C—500 milligrams twice daily, to be taken ten days to two weeks before and after surgery
- pain medication
- ophthalmic ointment (some physicians require this)
- antinausea medication
- oral antibiotics and/or ointment
- sleeping medication
- eye drops (artificial tears)—inform your physician if you are allergic to preservatives

  Be sure to follow your doctor's instructions.

PRE- AND POSTOPERATIVE INSTRUCTIONS

These suggestions are intended to make you more comfortable and help you heal. To learn more, turn to the section on recovery in this chapter. Your doctor may have different or additional instructions. Follow them to the letter.

- Stop smoking, discontinue the use of alcohol, and stop taking vitamin E and any medications containing aspirin or ibuprofen (two weeks pre- and postoperative is usually recommended). Check with your doctor regarding any other medications (including homeopathic/herbal products) that you are currently taking.
- Be sure you understand how and when to take/apply your prescriptions.
- Know how to cleanse the surgical areas the night before or the morning of your surgery.

- Do not have any food (including gum or mints) or drink (including water) for a minimum of six to eight hours prior to surgery. (Follow your surgical facility's preoperative instructions.)

- Have someone drive you to and from surgery.

- Have someone stay with you the first night after surgery (twenty-four hours, optimally).

- Dressings, if the procedure requires them, may be applied by the doctor or nurse immediately after the procedure.

- Follow directions regarding any ointments to be applied.

- Avoid straining during a bowel movement.

- Do not sunbathe or use tanning beds at least two weeks prior to surgery. (For optimal skin care and health, these should be avoided completely.) After surgery, if you must be in the sun, protect your eyelids.

- Avoid aerobic activity for at least three weeks after surgery.

- Do not drive for at least twenty-four hours after surgery and/or while taking pain medication.

- Wear sunglasses outside to protect your eyes from the light and wind.

- Keep the head elevated for at least the first week, optimally two weeks.

- Do not bend over for the first three weeks—if you must pick something up, squat with your knees bent.

- Lift nothing heavier than a small telephone book.

- Most doctors instruct that, for at least the first week, cold compresses should be applied for twenty minutes every hour for a minimum of forty-eight hours.

- Rest and relax for the first week. Your blood pressure must not be elevated.

- Do not wear your contact lenses after surgery until your doctor instructs you.

- Do not apply makeup until your doctor instructs you.

Recovery

Everyone heals differently. Healing is affected by your genetics, your physical and emotional well-being, whether you smoke and/or drink alcohol, your pain tolerance, the extent of the surgery, and how well you follow the doctor's instructions. Plan on approximately one to two weeks for the initial healing period.

POSTOPERATIVE PHYSICIAN APPOINTMENTS

Your doctor may want to see you the day after surgery. That activity alone may be all you want, or should do, that day. After your appointment, go home and rest. You may be given permission to shower that day or the next. Your sutures should be removed around the fifth to seventh day.

FIRST DAY POSTOPERATIVE

You may want to sleep the first day after surgery. Your eyes may be very swollen and bruised, and you may experience a mild burning sensation in your eyes.

SWELLING AND BRUISING

The swelling should lessen in the first few days, with some minor swelling remaining in the first weeks. You should expect to be black and blue. This may last, on the average, anywhere from five days to several weeks but should diminish daily. Remember—everyone heals differently. You may notice that the swelling and bruising drop (travel lower in the face) over the first few days. However, you can apply makeup (regular and/or camouflage) after the sutures are removed.

EYE SENSITIVITY

Your eyes may feel tired and sensitive to the light and you may experience a numb, tight, or itchy sensation. These should all be temporary.

COLD COMPRESSES

Cold compresses applied to the eye area may relieve some of the discomfort and can greatly reduce the swelling. These should be applied every hour for twenty minutes for a minimum of forty-eight hours (some doctors recommend seventy-two hours) after surgery. Ice should never be placed directly on the skin. Either use cold compresses or place a cloth between the ice bag and your skin. In some cases, your doctor may have instructed you *not* to use cold compresses. Follow your doctor's instructions.

BODY POSITION

It is important to keep your head elevated at all times for at least the first week. Surround yourself with pillows or sleep on a recliner if you must. Do not lie face down or bend over for the first three weeks. If you need to pick something up, squat with your knees bent. Do not pick up anything heavier than a small telephone book.

WALKING/EXERCISE

By the third day, you may be allowed to start walking around the house. Do not overdo it—listen to your body. If you feel tired, rest. By the fourth day, you can possibly resume some of your normal routine, except for strenuous activity or heavy lifting. Most physicians recommend that you wait a minimum of two to three weeks to resume aerobic exercise.

INCISION LINES

Your scars may remain red for four to six weeks and should gradually fade. Most scars become barely noticeable over time.

Pain

As with recovery times, pain tolerance is different for everyone. What one person may consider pain, another person may consider discomfort.

LEVEL OF PAIN/DISCOMFORT

Generally, with blepharoplasty there is minimal discomfort during the postoperative period. Some people experience absolutely no discomfort at all.

PAIN MEDICATION

Most discomfort can be controlled with pain medications you have been prescribed or Extra Strength Tylenol. You may find it necessary to take pain medication for the first day or two only.

Risks/Complications

Although problems are unlikely, you need to be aware of what can happen and what action you should take. Most risks/complications will be avoided if you

make an informed decision, choose a qualified physician, and follow your physician's instructions.

INFECTION

Pinkeye is rare, but any serious pain or heavy oozing should be reported immediately to the doctor. An infection can be treated with ophthalmic ointments or oral antibiotics.

BLEEDING

Bleeding is rare, but if it occurs, report it immediately to your doctor.

ECTROPION OR SCLERAL SHOW

An ectropion is a condition in which the lower eyelid pulls away or rolls out. With scleral show, the lower lid droops enough so that the white of the eye below the cornea shows. These conditions can occur if the skin under the eyes is tightened too much. Either condition may subside in three to six months as the skin relaxes. This condition most commonly occurs in patients who have had a transcutaneous (external incision) lower blepharoplasty.

DRY EYES

Dry eyes can be caused by lids unable to close completely (if too much skin is removed from the lid). This condition may be temporary until the eyelid stretches or could possibly be permanent. A cautious physician will err on the conservative side when removing upper eyelid skin. Additional skin can always be removed (called a touch-up) a few months postoperative via a simple procedure in the doctor's office. Dry eyes can also occur in up to 50 percent of patients when the lacrimal glands (tear glands) temporarily go into shock. Eye drops are used to treat this problem.

Note: Most doctors will not charge a professional fee for touch-ups performed within a certain time period after the original surgery. Ask your doctor what that time frame is.

*F*ace-Lift–Rhytidectomy

Rhytidectomy is specifically designed to help remove or lift sagging tissue that develops in the central and lower sections of the face, including the neck.

Different parts of the face age at different rates. Sagging jowls, cheeks, chin line, and neck can make a person appear old and tired. A face-lift can help rejuvenate a face and make it look more youthful and refreshed. As with any cosmetic surgery procedure, it is extremely important to be informed. Since the media does not always present all the options that are available, this section will help you be aware of the different techniques. Here are some important facts about rhytidectomy.

- Most patients are in their forties or older, but the procedure is occasionally performed on patients in their late thirties.

- A face-lift corrects sagging tissue of the jaw line and neck, not fine wrinkles, crow's feet, or the lines around the lips.

- A face-lift minimally affects the nasolabial folds (deep vertical creases that run between the nostrils and the corners of the mouth).

- Face-lifts do not affect the texture of the skin.

- Face-lifts are often performed in conjunction with blepharoplasty (eyelid surgery), rhinoplasty, brow/forehead lift, and collagen or fat injections.

Procedure

You must make some important decisions if you choose this procedure—the location of the incisions, technique, and your desired look. Educate yourself so that you can be a part of this decision-making process. The surgical options you choose may be determining factors in your physician selection. Remember that different doctors use different techniques and usually recommend the one(s) in which they are trained and experienced. In general, if you undergo a rhytidectomy, here's what you can expect.

While you are sitting, or under anesthesia, your doctor marks the areas of the face to be treated and indicates other landmarks (such as facial nerves).

ANESTHESIA

A face-lift can be performed under local anesthesia with intravenous sedation or under general anesthesia. The type of anesthesia is dependent on the extent of the procedure to be performed, the doctor's choice, and the patient's medical history or desires.

TECHNIQUES

A local anesthetic is injected into the areas to be treated. At this time, a small incision is placed underneath the chin if (1) fat is to be removed from under the chin via liposuction or (2) the bands of the neck (platysmal bands) are to be sutured together to improve that area (platysmaplasty). A chin implant can also be inserted through this incision.

Incisions are then made in front of the ears, following the natural folds and creases, into the ear canal, and back out under the earlobes and directly behind the ears into the scalp area. The incisions by the ears are placed differently on a man than they are on a woman because of the man's sideburns. A man's sideburns may end up narrower, closer to the ears, or at a different angle. Sometimes the incision will extend above the ears along the hairline to help improve the mid-face area.

The skin is lifted and separated from the underlying tissue. The sagging muscles, at this time, may be tightened—a SMAS (superficial musculo-aponeurotic system) face-lift. The skin is pulled back and the excess is trimmed. The incisions are closed with staples and/or sutures, and drains (plastic tubes to drain excess fluids) may be inserted behind the ears. The drains are usually removed twenty-four to forty-eight hours after surgery; the sutures will usually be removed in five to ten days, and the staples in about one to two weeks.

There are two additional techniques that some physicians may utilize in place of a face-lift for the early signs of aging.

STEPS IN THE FACE-LIFT PROCEDURE

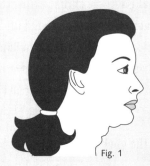

Fig. 1

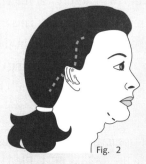

Fig. 2

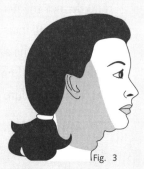

Fig. 3

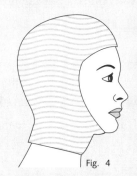

Fig. 4

A face-lift helps remove or lift sagging tissue that develops in the central and lower sections of the face, including the neck (Figure 1).

A small incision may be placed underneath the chin for liposuction, improvement of the platysmal bands, or placement of a chin implant. An incision is then made in front of the ears, following the natural folds and creases, into the ear canal, and back out under the earlobes and directly behind the ears into the scalp area. The incision may extend above the ears along the hairline to help improve the mid-face area (Figure 2).

The skin is lifted and separated from the underlying tissue, sagging muscles tightened, skin pulled back, and excess trimmed. Incisions are closed with staples and/or sutures, and drains (plastic tubes to drain excess fluids) may be inserted behind the ears (Figure 3).

A "mummy wrap" (sometimes as large as a football helmet) is applied, covering the entire head (Figure 4).

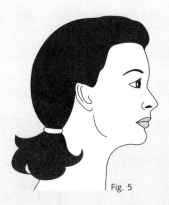

Fig. 5

Postoperatively, the areas addressed are firmer and more defined.

Chin Sling

The chin sling technique actually supports the platysmal bands in the neck and defines the neckline with a surgical material (Gore-Tex) that is inserted through small incisions behind the ears. This material is then threaded under the chin with the aid of another incision in the crease underneath the chin. The material is then sutured to the underlying tissue (periosteum) below each ear. This procedure is routinely done in combination with a platysmaplasty.

Pre-Jowl Implants

If there is evidence of tissue and/or bone loss in the jowl area, an implant that is as thin as a ribbon in the middle, thickening at each end, is inserted through an incision in the crease underneath the chin.

DRESSINGS

While you are still in the operating room, your doctor will apply a "mummy wrap" (sometimes as large as a football helmet) covering your entire head (there are a number of variations of dressings utilized). This dressing will be removed by the doctor or nurse a few days after surgery.

LENGTH OF PROCEDURE

A rhytidectomy will take approximately two and one-half to five hours, depending on the areas to be addressed.

Prior to Surgery

Before surgery, you and your doctor will first make several important decisions. Then you will prepare for surgery and be given prescriptions and instructions. The following sections will give you an overview of the process.

ASSESSMENT

Your physician will evaluate and assess the sagging skin of your face in conjunction with the laxity and position of the tissues. Your doctor may recommend a brow/forehead lift, eyelid surgery (blepharoplasty), chin or cheek implants, and/or laser resurfacing in combination with the face-lift to achieve the desired results. It is critical to have a thorough assessment. Be absolutely clear and in agreement with your doctor about your desired look.

PREOPERATIVE VISIT

You should be instructed to have certain lab tests, i.e., blood work, chest x-ray, EKG. (If you are also having a blepharoplasty, you may be required to have a thorough eye exam by an ophthalmologist). For the lab tests, you may go to your family doctor, a hospital facility, or an independent facility. The physician you have chosen may arrange for the performance of these tests.

You may sign all of your surgical consent forms, and be given pre- and post-operative instructions at this time. You should also be given your prescriptions for before and after surgery. Make sure that everything you and your physician have agreed on is stated on your consent form.

PRESCRIPTIONS

Some or all of these may be prescribed, in addition to others not listed.

- multivitamins—to be taken ten days to two weeks before and after surgery
- vitamin C—500 milligrams twice daily, to be taken ten days to two weeks before and after surgery
- pain medication
- antinausea medication
- oral antibiotics and/or ointment
- sleeping medication
- steroids (i.e., cortisone), to minimize swelling

Be sure to follow your doctor's instructions.

PRE- AND POSTOPERATIVE INSTRUCTIONS

These suggestions are intended to make you more comfortable and help you heal. To learn more, turn to the section on recovery in this chapter. Your doctor may have different or additional instructions. Follow them to the letter.

- Stop smoking, discontinue the use of alcohol, and stop taking vitamin E and any medications containing aspirin or ibuprofen (two weeks pre- and postoperative is usually recommended). Check with your doctor regarding any other medications (including homeopathic/herbal products) that you are currently taking.

- If you want to color your hair or have a permanent, do it a minimum of ten days prior to surgery. It will probably be about four to six weeks until you can color or have a permanent again.

- If you wear your hair short, do not have it cut prior to the procedure. In that way, the longer hair will help cover the incisions until they heal.

- Know how and when to take/apply your prescriptions.

- Know how to cleanse the surgical areas the night before or morning of your surgery.

- Do not have any food (including gum or mints) or drink (including water) for a minimum of six to eight hours prior to surgery. (Follow your surgical facility's preoperative instructions.)

- Have someone drive you to and from surgery.

- Have someone stay with you the first night after surgery (the first twenty-four hours, optimally).

- Dressings and/or drains, if these are required, will be applied by the doctor or nurse immediately after the procedure.

- Follow directions regarding any ointments to be applied and/or cleansing of incisions.

- Do not sunbathe or use tanning beds at least two weeks prior to surgery. (For optimal skin care and health, these should be avoided completely.) After surgery, if you must be in the sun, protect your face.

- Avoid aerobic activity for at least three weeks after surgery.

- Try not to drive or ride in a car for ten to fourteen days. You must avoid accidents to give the deep tissues adequate time to heal.

- Keep the head elevated above the level of your heart at all times for at least the first week, optimally two weeks.

- Do not turn or twist your neck—rotate your entire torso along with your head (as if you had a whiplash injury). After the second week, start gently rotating your head from side to side.

- For about a week, avoid excessive talking, laughing, and heavy chewing (stay on a soft diet). Brush your teeth gently.

- Do not bend over for the first three weeks—if you must pick something up, squat with your knees bent.

- Lift nothing heavier than a small telephone book.

- Do not rub your skin—be gentle for a minimum of a month.

- Expect some numbness in the areas treated for eight to twelve weeks. Be careful when using a hair dryer or curling iron, because you may not feel the heat.

- Your doctor may instruct you to apply cold compresses for twenty minutes every hour for a minimum of forty-eight hours.

- Rest and relax for the first week—your blood pressure must not be elevated.

- As your incisions start to heal, they may itch. Do not scratch them.

- Do not apply makeup until your doctor instructs you.

Recovery

Everyone heals differently. Healing is affected by your genetics, your physical and emotional well-being, whether you smoke and/or drink alcohol, your pain tolerance, the extent of the surgery, and how well you follow the doctor's instructions. Plan on approximately seven to ten days for the initial healing period.

POSTOPERATIVE PHYSICIAN APPOINTMENTS

Your doctor will probably want to see you the day after surgery. That activity alone may be all you will want to do, or should do, that day. If drains were inserted, they may be removed during this or the next appointment. After your appointment, go home and rest. Your next appointment should be within the next seven days. If a dressing was applied, this may be removed, and you may be given permission to shower that day or the next. You will have appointments to return to the doctor's office at about one week to ten days, again at two weeks, and then again in six weeks.

FIRST DAY POSTOPERATIVE

You may want to sleep the first day after surgery. You may experience some bruising and swelling. Because of the swelling, your face could appear very shiny.

Expect some numbness and a tight feeling in the treated areas for an average of eight to twelve weeks. This feeling can last up to a year.

BRUISING AND SWELLING

The swelling may shift over your face and neck area for the first few weeks. It will usually lessen daily, with some minor swelling remaining after the first few weeks. If there is increased swelling and/or bruising and tenderness, this may represent a hematoma (collection of blood) under the skin. Contact your physician immediately for evaluation. The bruising can last, on the average, anywhere from five days to several weeks but should diminish daily. Remember—everyone is different. Some patients have reported that the bruising dropped as low as the chest area. You can apply makeup (regular and/or camouflage) after the sutures/staples are removed.

NUMBNESS AND ITCHING

Expect some numbness in the central and lower sections of the face, including the neck, for at least eight to twelve weeks. Some patients have reported a level of numbness for up to a year or longer. However, the sensation tends to diminish over time. Also, if the incision sites itch, gently rub the areas—do not scratch them. Ask your doctor if you can apply some cream or ointment to relieve the itching, and only use what is recommended.

COLD COMPRESSES

Cold compresses applied to the face may relieve some of the discomfort and can greatly reduce the swelling. These should be applied every hour for twenty minutes for a minimum of forty-eight hours (some doctors recommend seventy-two hours) after surgery. Ice should never be placed directly on the skin. Either use cold compresses or place a cloth between the ice bag and your skin. In some cases, your doctor may have instructed you *not* to use cold compresses. Follow your doctor's instructions.

BODY POSITION

It is important that you keep your head elevated at all times for at least the first week, optimally two weeks. Sleep on a recliner or prop yourself up with pillows. Under no circumstances should you lie face down or bend over for the first three weeks. If you need to pick something up, squat with your knees bent;

and do not pick up anything heavier than a small telephone book. Avoid excessive talking, laughing, or chewing for the first week. For the first two weeks, if you have to turn your head, rotate your entire body with your head.

WALKING/EXERCISE

By the third day, you may be allowed to start walking around the house. Do not overdo it—listen to your body. If you feel tired, rest. By the fourth day, you can possibly resume some of your normal routine, except for strenuous activity or heavy lifting. Most physicians recommend that you wait a minimum of two to three weeks to resume aerobic exercise.

SKIN CHANGES

Your facial skin may go through some changes in the first few weeks—it may break out or become dry or oily. This is only temporary. The cause is a combination of trauma and the anesthesia.

INCISION LINES

Your scars may remain red for four to six weeks and should gradually fade. Most scars become barely noticeable over time. If the scars become raised or thickened as well as red, then notify your physician immediately. This may represent hypertrophic scarring, which can be treated. There also may be temporary hair loss in the incision area(s), but this usually improves within four to six months.

Pain

As with recovery times, pain tolerance is different for everyone. What one person may consider pain, another person may consider discomfort.

LEVEL OF PAIN/DISCOMFORT

Generally, with a face-lift there is minimal to moderate discomfort during the postoperative period. Some people experience absolutely no discomfort at all.

PAIN MEDICATION

Most discomfort can be controlled with pain medications you have been prescribed or Extra Strength Tylenol. You may find it necessary to take pain medication for the first day or two only.

Risks/Complications

Although problems are unlikely, you need to be aware of what can happen and what action you should take. Most risks/complications will be avoided if you make an informed decision, choose a qualified physician, and follow your physician's instructions.

HEMATOMA

A hematoma, a collection of blood or fluid beneath the skin, is unlikely. However, it can usually be treated by drainage with a needle or with compression, or it may require a return to the operating room.

NERVE DAMAGE

Loss of sensation and/or movement of the face is usually temporary.

HYPERTROPHIC SCARRING

Report any signs of hypertrophic scarring immediately to your doctor; it can be treated if caught early. (See "Definitions of Scarring/Skin Changes," page 56.)

SKIN SLOUGH

The outer layer of skin may die and then subsequently peel. There is an increased risk of this condition in smokers or diabetics.

Hair Restoration

A variety of options are utilized to restore a natural hairline. A person may become bald because of illness, poor nutrition, chemotherapy, or most commonly, genetics. A full head of hair can certainly make a person look more youthful. Because many companies feed on people's desperation and the media does not always present the options that are available, this section will help you be aware of the different techniques. Here are some interesting facts about hair restoration.

- Rogaine (minoxidil) may be recommended before and after hair transplantation. Many doctors feel that it increases the blood supply to the scalp, thus "fertilizing" the regrowth of hair.

- The newest antibaldness drug, Propecia, helps regrow hair and prevent more from falling out by suppressing a testosterone-related hormone, dihyrotestosterone, or DHT, that shrinks hair follicles. Many studies have found greater results with a regime of Propecia and Rogaine. However, there are questions regarding Propecia's long-term side effects.

- Today's micrografting techniques achieve a natural look when performed by a skilled and experienced physician/technician. It is an art.

- The area of baldness can be reduced via the method of scalp reduction.

- Hair-bearing portions of the scalp can be rotated (lifted) to the balding area.

- Hair transplantation can be performed in conjunction with many other plastic surgery procedures.

- If a patient does not quit smoking for a minimum of two days before and five days after surgery, there is a chance that the grafts will not "take."

- Baldness is a progressive condition.

Procedure

You must make some important decisions if you choose this procedure—technique(s) to be performed, location of incisions, and your desired look. Educate yourself so that you can be a part of this decision-making process. The surgical options you choose may be determining factors in your physician selection. Remember that different doctors use different techniques and usually recommend the one(s) in which they are trained and experienced. In general, if you undergo hair restoration, here's what you can expect.

ANESTHESIA

Hair transplantation (grafting) can be performed under local anesthesia and oral sedation. Other procedures such as scalp reduction and scalp lifting (scalp rotation) may require local anesthesia with intravenous sedation. The type of anesthesia is dependent on the extent of procedure to be performed, the doctor's choice, and the patient's medical history or desires.

TECHNIQUES

A patient currently has several options to choose from.

Hair Grafting or Transplantation

A strip of hair-bearing scalp (the size is determined by the number of grafts to be transplanted) from the back of the head (never at the neckline) is removed. The incision of this donor site is then closed with staples or sutures. The hair-bearing strip is divided into micro- and minigrafts. Great care is taken to maintain the integrity of the follicles. The number of hairs in each graft may vary from one for the hairline to three or four (sometimes more) for the crown of the head.

The harvested grafts are then placed into tiny incisions that have been cut at the angle of the hair growth in the bald areas of the scalp. The incisions do not generally require sutures.

While you are still in the operating facility, your doctor may apply a "turban" dressing, which could remain in place until the next day or until your first postoperative appointment. Initial recovery time is approximately two to three days. If a lot of frontal (hairline) work has been done, it is extremely important to take it easy for seventy-two hours. Otherwise, there could be extreme swelling, which could take approximately five to seven days to dissipate.

The transplanted hair falls out in approximately ten days to two weeks, followed by regrowth of hair in two to four months. Hair transplantation may require a minimum of two to three sessions.

The amount of time for each session of hair transplantation is dependent on the number of hairs to be transplanted. This is a time intensive procedure (a large area to be transplanted could take most of the day).

Scalp Reduction

A section of the bald area is removed. The incision is then sutured or stapled. Your doctor may determine that this technique can be performed a second time. The reduction method greatly reduces, and in some cases eliminates, the bald area. If there is still an area of baldness, hair transplantation can then be performed, if desired. A "turban" dressing may be applied after surgery and may remain in place for about twenty-four hours. Recovery time is approximately three to five days.

Scalp Lifting or Rotation

A section of the bald area is removed. A section of hair-bearing scalp is then lifted and rotated to the bald area and stapled or sutured into place. The donor site is also stapled or sutured. A "turban" dressing may be applied after surgery and may remain in place for twenty-four hours. Recovery time is approximately three to five days.

Extenders/Expanders

Two types of extenders are currently available. A scalp extender is a device made of Silastic (elastic material) with a small-toothed comb at each end. It is placed under the bald area to loosen the scalp and stretch the hair-bearing areas. A scalp reduction and/or hair transplantation may be done in conjunction with the placement of the scalp extender. The extender is left in place for four to six weeks, depending on the elasticity of the scalp. Upon removal, a scalp reduction is performed to reduce the area of baldness. Recovery time is approximately three to five days, during which time there may be mild to moderate discomfort. Most physicians recommend that the prescribed pain medication be taken for the first three to five days to minimize discomfort.

STEPS IN THE HAIR RESTORATION PROCEDURE

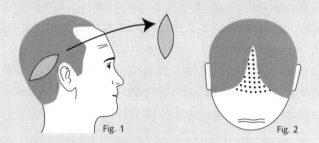

Fig. 1

Fig. 2

Hair Grafting or Transplantation: A strip of hair-bearing scalp from the back of the head is removed (Figure 1). The incision of this donor site is closed with staples or sutures. This strip is divided into micro- and minigrafts. The harvested grafts are placed into tiny incisions that have been cut at the angle of the hair growth in the bald areas of the scalp (Figure 2). The incisions do not generally require sutures.

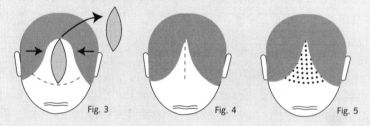

Fig. 3

Fig. 4

Fig. 5

Scalp Reduction: A section of the bald area is removed (Figure 3), and the incision is sutured or stapled (Figure 4). If there is still an area of baldness, hair transplantation can then be performed (Figure 5).

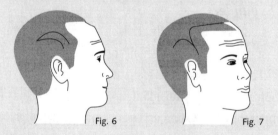

Fig. 6

Fig. 7

Scalp Lifting/Rotation: A section of the bald area is removed. A section of hair-bearing scalp is then lifted and rotated to the bald area and sutured into place (Figures 6 and 7). The donor site is also stapled or sutured.

A tissue expander is a balloon-like device placed under the hair-bearing scalp (usually at the back of the head). The expander is enlarged with saline weekly for a period of one to two months. At that time, a scalp reduction or lift can be performed. This method is not used often because of the noticeable bulge as the extender is filled. Recovery time is approximately three to five days.

Prior to Surgery

Before surgery, you and your doctor will first make several important decisions. Then you will prepare for surgery and be given prescriptions and instructions. The following sections will give you an overview of the process.

ASSESSMENT

Your physician should diagnose the cause of your hair loss via a thorough evaluation and possibly some testing. Your doctor may discuss the different options available to you and should then work with you to design a plan that addresses your specific needs. It is critical to have a thorough assessment. Be absolutely clear and in agreement with your doctor about your desired look and goals.

PREOPERATIVE VISIT

You should be instructed to have certain lab tests, i.e., blood work, chest x-ray, EKG. For the lab tests, you may go to your family doctor, a hospital facility, or an independent facility. The physician you have chosen may arrange for the performance of these tests.

You may sign all of your surgical consent forms and be given pre- and postoperative instructions at this time. You should also be given your prescriptions for before and after surgery. Make sure that everything you and your physician have agreed on is stated on your consent form.

PRESCRIPTIONS

Some or all of these may be prescribed, in addition to others not listed.

- multivitamins—to be taken ten days to two weeks before and after surgery
- vitamin C—500 milligrams twice daily, to be taken ten days to two weeks before and after surgery
- pain medication

- antinausea medication
- oral antibiotics and/or ointment
- sleeping medication

Be sure to follow your doctor's instructions.

PRE- AND POSTOPERATIVE INSTRUCTIONS

These suggestions are intended to make you more comfortable and help you heal. To learn more, turn to the section on recovery in this chapter. Your doctor may have different or additional instructions. Follow them to the letter. The recovery time for hair transplants is minimal (approximately two to three days). The more advanced procedures (scalp reduction, scalp lifting) may require three to five days.

- Stop smoking, discontinue the use of alcohol, and stop taking vitamin E and any medications containing aspirin or ibuprofen (two weeks pre- and postoperative is usually recommended). Check with your doctor regarding any other medications (including homeopathic/herbal products) that you are currently taking.

- If you want to color your hair or have a permanent, do it a minimum of ten days prior to surgery. It is generally a minimum of four to six weeks until you can color or have a permanent again (ask your doctor).

- Grow your hair a little longer than usual before the procedure. In that way, the longer hair will help cover the incision(s). The doctor should only cut hair at the donor site (which is excised and removed).

- Be sure you understand how and when to take/apply your prescriptions.

- Know how to cleanse the surgical areas the night before or morning of your surgery.

- If undergoing intravenous sedation or general anesthesia, do not have any food (including gum or mints) or drink (including water) for a minimum of six to eight hours prior to surgery (follow your surgical facility's preoperative instructions).

- Have someone drive you to and from surgery.

- Have someone stay with you the first night after surgery (the first twenty-four hours, optimally).
- Dressings, if the procedure requires them, should be applied by the doctor or nurse immediately after the procedure.
- Follow directions regarding any ointments to be applied.
- If your doctor instructs you to use cold compresses, apply them for twenty minutes every hour for a minimum of forty-eight hours.
- Do not sunbathe or use tanning beds at least two weeks prior to surgery. (For optimal skin care and health, these activities should be avoided completely.) After surgery, your scalp must be protected from exposure to the sun.
- Avoid strenuous or aerobic activity for at least three weeks after surgery.
- Do not drive for at least twenty-four hours after surgery and/or while taking pain medication.
- Keep the head elevated at all times for at least the first week, optimally two weeks.
- Do not bend over for the first three weeks—if you must pick something up, squat with your knees bent.
- Lift nothing heavier than a small telephone book.
- When using a hair dryer or curling iron, use a cool or warm setting—you don't want to jeopardize the incisions or damage the new hairs.
- Brush or comb your hair very carefully so that you do not disturb the staples or sutures at the donor site, or the grafts.
- Rest and relax for one to two days for hair transplantation, three to five days for more extensive hair restoration procedures.

Recovery

Everyone heals differently. Healing is affected by your genetics, your physical and emotional well-being, whether you smoke and/or drink alcohol, your pain tolerance, the extent of the surgery, and how well you follow the doctor's instructions. For hair transplantation, you should plan on approximately two to three days for the initial healing period. For more extensive procedures, plan on three to five days.

POSTOPERATIVE PHYSICIAN APPOINTMENTS

Your doctor may want to see you the day after surgery. That activity alone may be all you will want, or should do, that day. If a dressing was applied, this may be removed and your head shampooed. After your appointment, go home and rest. You may be given permission to shower that day or the next. You need to schedule an appointment to return to the doctor's office in about one week to ten days.

FIRST DAY POSTOPERATIVE

Take it easy for a couple of days. There may be swelling and numbness in the grafting and donor sites.

SWELLING

The swelling should lessen in the first few days, with some minor swelling remaining in the first weeks. Remember—everyone is different. If you have had extensive frontal (hairline) work, the swelling could drop to the brow and eye area and become extreme. In some patients, the eyes may swell shut. Such swelling could then take five to seven days to dissipate.

COLD COMPRESSES

Cold compresses applied to the scalp area (only if your doctor has instructed you to do so) may relieve some of the discomfort and can greatly reduce the swelling. These should be applied every hour for twenty minutes for a minimum of forty-eight hours (some doctors recommend seventy-two hours) after surgery. Ice should never be placed directly on the skin. Either use cold compresses or place a cloth between the ice bag and your skin. In some cases, your doctor may have instructed you *not* to use cold compresses. Follow your doctor's instructions.

INCISIONS AND CARE OF SCALP

You should be given specific instructions concerning shampooing your scalp and cleaning the incisions (when, how, and what products to use). In addition, some doctors recommend "saline soaks" (application of saline-soaked gauze pads). If you have sutures/staples, they may be removed at your appointment one week to ten days after the procedure. Your scars may remain red for four to six weeks and will gradually fade. Most scars become barely noticeable over time.

BODY POSITION

It is imperative that you keep your head elevated at all times for at least the first week. Surround yourself with pillows or sleep on a recliner. Under no circumstances should you lie face down or bend over for the first two weeks. If you need to pick something up, squat with your knees bent. And do not pick up anything heavier than a small telephone book.

WALKING/EXERCISE

By the third or fifth day (depending on the procedure performed), you may be allowed to resume your normal routine, except for strenuous activity or heavy lifting. Do not overdo it—listen to your body. If you feel tired, rest. Most physicians recommend that you wait a minimum of two to three weeks to resume aerobic exercise or weightlifting.

Pain

As with recovery times, pain tolerance is different for everyone. What one person may consider pain, another person may consider discomfort.

LEVEL OF PAIN/DISCOMFORT

Generally, with hair transplantation there is minimal discomfort during the postoperative period. Some people experience absolutely no discomfort at all.

PAIN MEDICATION

Most discomfort can be controlled with pain medications you have been prescribed or Extra Strength Tylenol. You may find it necessary to take pain medication for the first day or two only, depending on the procedures performed.

Risks/Complications

Although problems are unlikely, you need to be aware of what can happen and what action you should take. Most risks/complications will be avoided if you

make an informed decision, choose a qualified physician, and follow your physician's instructions.

HEMATOMA

A hematoma, a collection of blood or fluid beneath the scalp, is unlikely. However, it can be treated by drainage with a needle or with compression.

NERVE DAMAGE

Loss of sensation and/or movement is usually temporary.

HYPERTROPHIC SCARRING

Report any signs of hypertrophic scarring immediately to your doctor; it can be treated if caught early. (See "Definitions of Scarring/Skin Changes," page 56.)

$\mathcal{L}$aser Resurfacing

L aser resurfacing works by removing the top layer(s) of skin, resulting in an improvement of fine lines, wrinkles, skin tone, and irregular pigmentation that are unaffected by a face-lift.

The word "laser" is an acronym for *light amplification by stimulated emission of radiation.* A laser beam can be adjusted so that it destroys a specific organic target. Different lasers are used to treat fine wrinkles, scars, tattoos, spider veins, freckles, age spots, rosacea (a chronic acne-like condition of the facial skin), and birthmarks. The use of lasers and laser resurfacing is booming. That boom has attracted many newcomers to the business. As a result, laser resurfacing is being performed by physicians who may or may not have the proper training and experience. For this reason, it is even more important for you to be totally informed. Here are some interesting facts about laser resurfacing.

- A laser works best on the fine lines around the eyes and mouth.
- Some lines will reappear, but they will be less obvious.
- The fairer the skin, the less potential for pigmentation problems.
- The pulsed laser vaporizes the top few layers of skin and shrinks the underlying collagen tissue, resulting in a tightening of the skin.
- The laser has a computer attached to it so that the depth of the tissue removal can be controlled. This is crucial.
- The beam of most physicians' lasers is pulsed (or regulated) so that excess heat does not build up in the surrounding tissues.

Procedure

Many patients choose laser resurfacing to turn back the hands of time either as a procedure by itself or in conjunction with surgical facial procedures because of its tightening effect (the skin actually shrinks). Your physician will guide you as to which laser and procedures will accomplish your desired goals. Many physicians nowadays are utilizing the erbium laser instead of medium chemical peels and the CO_2 laser as a replacement for deep chemical peels and dermabrasion. They feel that they have more control over the depth of the peel with the laser. Make sure that your physician has had extensive experience in laser resurfacing, not just a weekend course. If not, find another physician. In general, if you undergo laser resurfacing, here's what you can expect.

TYPES OF RESURFACING LASERS

Currently, two types of lasers for resurfacing are available. They can be used alone or in conjunction with each other. Which kind you choose will be determined by what you wish to accomplish.

CO_2 Laser

The laser beam passes through a chamber filled with carbon dioxide. It generates extremely high temperatures. For deep wrinkles, the result is similar to a deep chemical peel or dermabrasion. This procedure requires an anesthetic. Pinkness usually lasts from one to six months. The healing period can be lengthy and complex. Makeup can usually be applied between seven and ten days after treatment.

Erbium Laser

This laser produces a shallower laser area and less heat and has a light, smoothing effect for fine lines and pigmentation. The procedure is similar to a light-to-medium peel, depending on how many passes are made over the surface. It may not require anesthetic (a topical anesthetic or injection may be necessary in delicate areas). The erbium laser has been used on the delicate neck area and the backs of the hands. This laser also has been used successfully on darker skins. Blisters do not form, and the recuperation period is shorter and less complex.

The following information pertains to deep laser resurfacing via the CO_2 laser, sometimes referred to as the "Ultra Pulse."

ANESTHESIA

If the area to be treated is small, such as around the eyes or mouth, a local anesthetic may be used. However, intravenous sedation or general anesthesia is generally used for full-face laser resurfacing. The type of anesthesia is dependent on the area(s) to be treated, the doctor's choice, and the patient's medical history or desires.

TECHNIQUES

The patient is placed in a reclining or lying position. The face is cleansed to remove all makeup and oils, an antiseptic solution is applied, and the areas to be laser peeled are marked. The patient's eyes are then covered with thick, moistened gauze pads or metal shields to prevent damage, and the anesthesia is administered.

The physician moves the laser across the skin, working on one small area at a time. If full face resurfacing is not being performed, the depth of the laser peel should get progressively shallower (sometimes referred to as "feathering") toward the edges of the area being treated. In this manner, the treated area(s) blend with the rest of the skin. The sensation is sometimes described as that of a rubber band snapping against the skin. The patient may hear a popping and fizz as the laser is applied to the skin, and a vacuum is used to remove the vaporized skin cells. A varying number of passes are made, depending on the depth of the wrinkles, the skin type, and the laser settings.

DRESSINGS

Two different techniques are used for protecting the face after the procedure: some physicians apply a special dressing that stays on for approximately a week; others apply an antiseptic ointment, which may be replaced in a few days with a petroleum jelly product.

LENGTH OF PROCEDURE

The procedure can take anywhere from fifteen minutes for small areas to forty-five minutes or longer for full-face laser resurfacing.

Prior to Surgery

Before surgery, you and your doctor will first make several important decisions. Then you will prepare for surgery and be given prescriptions and instructions. The following sections will give you an overview of the process.

ASSESSMENT

Your physician should discuss with you the areas you want to have laser resurfaced and should evaluate your skin type, the degree of sun damage, and the depth and location of wrinkles. The muscle tone of your lower eyelids should also be assessed to prevent the complication of an ectropion (drooping lower eyelid) that may occur from the tightening effect of the lower eyelid skin. Your doctor may recommend a canthopexy (eyelid tightening procedure) prior to the resurfacing.

AVOIDANCE OF SUN

All patients are at risk for hyperpigmentation, a darkening of the skin. Certain skin types are at higher risk than others. Many doctors prescribe skin lightening creams that inhibit the formation of melanin (pigment). The doctor should also strongly warn patients to avoid the sun after surgery for a minimum of three months. Even sunlight through a window must be strictly avoided.

MEDICAL HISTORY DISCLOSURE

If you will be undergoing any type of facial peel—chemical peel, dermabrasion, or laser resurfacing—it is imperative that you tell your doctor if you have a history of cold sores, shingles, or herpes infections because these procedures can reactivate the virus. Many doctors routinely prescribe an oral antiviral medication. It is also extremely important to tell your doctor if you have taken any acne medication (such as Accutane) in the past year, or if you have any connective tissue disease, e.g., lupus, scleroderma.

PREOPERATIVE VISIT

You should be instructed to have certain lab tests, i.e., blood work, chest x-ray, EKG. You may go to your family doctor, a hospital facility, or an independent facility. The physician you have chosen may arrange for the performance of these tests.

You may sign all of your surgical consent forms and will be given pre- and postoperative instructions at this time. You should also be given your prescriptions for before and after surgery. Make sure that everything you and your physician have agreed on is stated on your consent form.

PRESCRIPTIONS

Some or all of these may be prescribed, in addition to others not listed.

- antiviral medication—some physicians may prescribe this, whether or not you have a previous history of herpes infections
- Retin-A/alpha-hydroxy acids/topical vitamin solutions/topical steroids— some doctors pretreat their patients because these products aid cell rejuvenation and exfoliation
- skin lightening creams—some doctors pretreat to prevent the possible temporary complication of skin darkening (transient hyperpigmentation)
- multivitamins—to be taken ten days to two weeks before and after surgery
- vitamin C—500 milligrams twice daily, to be taken ten days to two weeks before and after surgery
- pain medication
- antinausea medication
- oral antibiotics and/or ointment
- sleeping medication
- steroids (i.e., cortisone—topical and/or oral)

Be sure to follow your doctor's instructions.

PRE- AND POSTOPERATIVE INSTRUCTIONS

These suggestions are intended to make you more comfortable and help you heal. To learn more, turn to the section on recovery in this chapter. Your doctor may have different or additional instructions. Follow them to the letter.

- Stop smoking, discontinue the use of alcohol, and stop taking vitamin E and any medications containing aspirin or ibuprofen (two weeks pre- and postoperative is usually recommended). Check with your doctor regarding any other medications (including homeopathic/herbal products) that you are currently taking.
- Purchase cotton gloves to wear at night, especially if you are prone to scratching yourself while sleeping.
- Be sure you understand how and when to take/apply your prescriptions.

- Know how to cleanse the surgical areas the night before or morning of your surgery.

- Do not have any food (including gum or mints) or drink (including water) for a minimum of six to eight hours prior to surgery. (Follow your surgical facility's preoperative instructions.)

- Have someone drive you to and from surgery.

- Have someone stay with you for at least the first night after surgery (the first twenty-four hours, optimally).

- Dressings, if the procedure requires them, should be applied by the doctor or nurse immediately after the procedure.

- Keep the head elevated.

- Follow directions regarding any ointments to be applied.

- Do not sunbathe or use tanning beds at least six weeks prior to surgery and three to six months after surgery depending on your healing. Otherwise the pigmentation of your skin may change permanently. (Optimally, for skin care and health, these should be avoided completely.)

- Avoid aerobic activity for at least three weeks after surgery.

- Do not drive for at least twenty-four hours after surgery and/or while taking pain medication.

Recovery

Everyone heals differently. Healing is affected by your genetics, your physical and emotional well-being, whether you smoke and/or drink alcohol, your pain tolerance, the extent of the surgery, and how well you follow the doctor's instructions. Plan on approximately two full weeks before you will be able, or want, to go out in public (usually with some camouflage makeup for redness).

COMPLEX HEALING

Healing from laser resurfacing is complex. It requires a demanding regimen of home care and strict adherence to your doctor's pre- and postoperative instructions.

Your skin can be abnormally susceptible to infection for several weeks after the operation. Candida (yeast), herpes, and staphylococcus infections are particular dangers; all can cause skin changes that may result in a scar. Call your doctor instantly if you develop any signs of infection such as a high fever, severe localized pain, or swelling (after the initial swelling has subsided), or any kind of blistering or discharge, other than the clear oozing typical of the first few days.[1]

DRESSINGS/OINTMENT

Depending on the technique your doctor employs, your face could be coated either with an antibiotic ointment, petroleum jelly, or with a thin dressing that maintains moisture (your face may be wrapped like a mummy). Your doctor may replace the dressing the day after your surgery. The dressing generally stays in place until the skin has built up a new surface layer of cells. This usually takes an average of five to seven days.

FIRST DAY POSTOPERATIVE

After surgery, the areas that have been treated could be very sensitive and red and may start to swell immediately. Keep your head elevated at all times. Your eyes may be swollen almost shut, and it may be uncomfortable to open your mouth. It is best to minimize the movement of your mouth in the first few weeks of healing. The swelling usually starts to go down in two to three days. Within twenty-four hours your skin will start to ooze a watery, yellowish serum.

PHYSICIAN INSTRUCTIONS

There are a number of different techniques that doctors employ at this stage to prevent or minimize the formation of crusts. *Follow your doctor's instructions to the letter.* Some doctors instruct the patient to wash the face a number of times during the day and then apply an ointment or petroleum jelly; some advise the application of cold compresses to dissolve the crusts; others instruct that you apply an ointment or petroleum jelly and/or apply cold compresses if a dressing has been applied on your face. If you are instructed to apply

---

[1] Tina Alster, M.D., and Lydia Preston, *Cosmetic Laser Surgery*, (Brooklyn: Alliance Publications, 1997).

cold compresses, it is imperative that something is between the compress and your skin—either a washcloth or the dressings. *Do not pick any crusts—this could cause scarring.* Your doctor may schedule another postoperative appointment for the third or fourth day. At that time, if you have any stubborn areas of crusting, these may be soaked or steamed.

Remember—do not apply anything to the treated areas except what is recommended or prescribed by your doctor. If you notice intense redness in one area and feel an underlying hardness or stiffness in that area, notify your doctor right away—you could be developing a hypertrophic (raised) scar. Unless treated early, a permanent scar can form.

FIRST WEEK TO TWO WEEKS POSTOPERATIVE

The oozing and crusting can require approximately one to two weeks to heal. Once new surface cells have built up (an average of five to seven days), the redness and sensitivity should lessen, and you can generally apply makeup. As your skin heals, it may feel drier than normal and begin to flake or appear chapped. You may also break out in bumps and pimples or may begin to itch. At three to four weeks, the treated areas may darken and turn brown (transient hyperpigmentation). All of these can be treated, so notify your doctor immediately.

ITCHING

Itching is common during the first week to three weeks. Do not scratch. You may want to wear cotton gloves during the night, especially if you are prone to scratching yourself while sleeping. Some physicians may prescribe medication for the itching.

SWELLING AND REDNESS

The swelling should dissipate over the first few weeks. However, your skin could feel tight and dry for about six weeks. The redness should turn to pink, and it can then take (on average) up to three months for the pinkness to fade, maybe longer. Remember—everyone's healing time is different.

Pain

As with recovery times, pain tolerance is different for everyone. What one person may consider pain, another person may consider discomfort.

LEVEL OF PAIN/DISCOMFORT

Generally, with laser resurfacing the level of pain can be minimal to extreme (much of it is dependent on your adherence to the doctor's pre- and postoperative instructions).

PAIN MEDICATION

Most pain or discomfort can be controlled with pain medications you have been prescribed or Extra Strength Tylenol. You may find it necessary to take pain medication for the first day or two only. The dressing and/or ointment minimize, and in some cases eliminate, any discomfort.

Risks/Complications

Although problems are unlikely, you need to be aware of what can happen and what action you should take. Most risks/complications will be avoided if you make an informed decision, choose a qualified physician, and follow your physician's instructions.

SCARRING

Scarring could occur if the skin becomes infected. It is of utmost importance to take/apply antibiotics and/or antiviral drugs your doctor has prescribed.

DISCOLORATION

Blotchy patches (pigmentation changes) may appear, especially on darker complexions. This is temporary if treated with lightening creams as prescribed by your doctor.

ECTROPION OR SCLERAL SHOW

An ectropion is a condition in which the lower eyelid pulls away or rolls out. With scleral show, the lower lid droops enough so that the white of the eye below the cornea shows. These conditions can occur if the skin under the eyes tightens too much. Either condition may subside in three to six months as the skin relaxes. This condition most commonly occurs in patients who have had a transcutaneous (external incision) lower blepharoplasty.

CHANGE IN TEXTURE OF THE SKIN

Pores may be clogged. This problem usually clears up on its own or may need to be treated. Consult with your physician's skin care specialist.

$\mathcal{L}$iposuction

$\mathcal{L}$iposuction is the suction-assisted removal of fat cells from certain areas of the body. Areas can include the face, neck, chin, upper arms, breasts, abdomen, hips, buttocks, thighs, knees, calves, and ankles.

Liposuction is the most common cosmetic surgery procedure performed today and has the highest satisfaction rate among patients. Because of the popularity of this procedure, everyone wants to get on the bandwagon. As a result, liposuction is being performed by physicians who may or may not have the proper training and experience. For this reason, it is even more important for you to be totally informed. Here are some interesting facts about liposuction.

- The operation and recovery are generally associated with minimal discomfort.

- Liposuction cannot remove cellulite.

- Intravenous sedation with local anesthesia is generally used.

- Liposuction may be used in conjunction with mammaplasty (breast reduction).

- It may be used in the treatment of enlarged male breasts (gynecomastia).

- Excess fat is broken up and vacuumed out through a tube called a cannula.

- Cannulas are narrower today, so incisions are very small (sometimes do not even require sutures).

- Different sizes of cannulas are used on different parts of the body.

Procedure

Liposuction techniques have changed dramatically in the last few years. There is little or no blood loss with today's standard technique (tumescent liposuction)

217

so that more fat can be removed than in years past. However, liposuction is not a cure for overeating or an excuse for not keeping fit. Fat can return to the treated areas if you gain weight. Make sure that your physician has had extensive experience in liposuction, not just a weekend course. If not, find another physician. If you undergo liposuction, here's what you can expect.

ANESTHESIA

Liposuction is usually performed under intravenous sedation with local anesthesia, but some doctors perform it under general or epidural (spinal block) anesthesia. The type of anesthesia is dependent on the areas to be treated, the doctor's choice, and the patient's medical history or desires.

TECHNIQUES

Your doctor should use a special marker to carefully mark the areas to be treated. A topographic map is created on your body of areas to be treated by drawing concentric circles. The highest number of concentric circles indicates the areas with the greatest amount of fat.

Tumescent Liposuction—The Standard Technique Used Today

This technique reduces blood loss dramatically and results in less bruising, less fatigue, and less discomfort. Swelling also diminishes faster. A solution of epinephrine (which constricts the blood vessels) and a diluted anesthetic are injected into the fat. Since there is very little blood loss, more fat can be removed than in the past. Additionally, because the anesthetic remains in the tissues for eighteen to twenty-four hours after the surgery, there is much less postoperative discomfort.

Incisions are made in appropriate locations on the body, depending on the areas to be addressed. The incisions are very small (usually one-quarter inch long) and placed, as much as possible, in the natural creases. The epinephrine-anesthetic solution is injected through the incisions, and then the cannula is inserted. As the fat is extracted, a sense of movement or pressure may be felt (described by some patients as the same feeling as a heavy, deep-muscle massage). Upon completion, the incisions are sutured, if necessary, and dressed.

Ultrasonic Assisted Liposuction (UAL)

The main function of UAL is to liquefy fat. There are two methods available to accomplish this, both used in conjunction with the tumescent technique.

In external UAL, a stylus emitting ultrasonic sound waves is passed over the areas (on the surface of the skin) to be treated to warm the fat. The fat is then "vacuumed" out via a cannula. Some physicians feel that the external UAL also helps distribute the local anesthetic more evenly into the tissues. However, there is currently no data to prove or support this.

Internal UAL is actually two techniques. In the two-stage technique, a probe emitting ultrasonic sound waves is inserted, and the fat is liquefied. The fat is then vacuumed out via a cannula. Because of the possibility of greater complications with this technique, the physician requires additional specialized training. Verify your physician's certificates in this procedure. In the one-stage internal UAL technique, a special cannula (a combination of cannula and probe) emitting ultrasonic sound waves is inserted. As the fat is liquefied, it is vacuumed.

Advantages of UAL include the following:

- Results may be better in areas to be treated that are scarred from previous surgeries.

- Results may be better on men because their fat is more fibrous (UAL helps break up the fibers, making extraction of the fat easier).

- Results may be better on certain areas of women that contain fibrous fat, such as the back.

- Skin retraction may be better.

The following are disadvantages of UAL:

- The cannula/probe is bigger, requiring larger incisions and sutures.

- The procedure takes a greater amount of time than traditional liposuction.

- The ultrasonic waves are emitted through the entire probe/cannula, not just the tip. As a result, the potential for tissue burns exists.

- UAL may cause "tunnels" (depressions).

- UAL may result in a seroma, a pocket of fluid that collects under the skin. This can be drained.

Some physicians feel that, in the hands of an experienced doctor, this is a very beneficial and useful technique. However, according to other physicians,

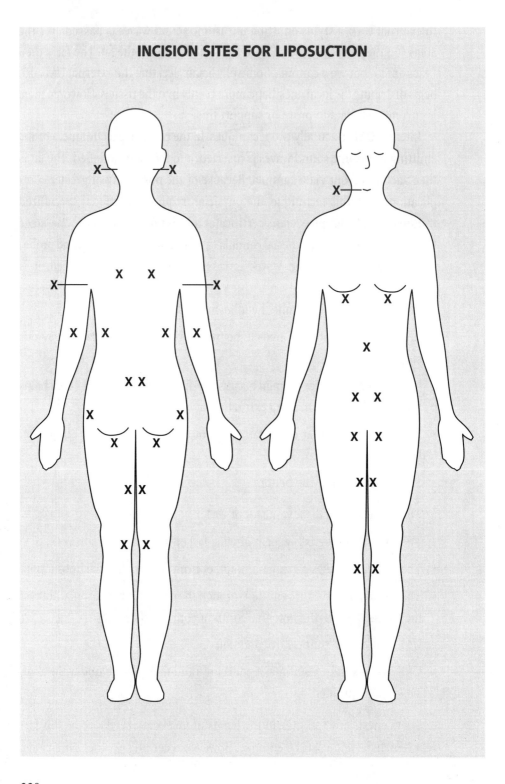

INCISION SITES FOR LIPOSUCTION

there is still debate as to the benefits of ultrasonic assisted liposuction (UAL). Some feel that the potential complications outweigh the advantages.

DRESSINGS

While you are still in the operating room, pads/dressings may be placed on the incision sites, and a restrictive garment or elastic tape may be applied. These mold and hold the skin in place and aid it in adhering to the underlying tissue. They also help in reducing swelling and bleeding.

LENGTH OF PROCEDURE

This is a one- to five-hour procedure (depending on the areas to be treated) and is usually performed in an outpatient surgery center.

Prior to Surgery

Before surgery, you and your doctor will first make several important decisions. Then you will prepare for surgery and be given prescriptions and instructions. The following sections will give you an overview of the process.

ASSESSMENT

Your physician should discuss with you what you do not like about your body. The physician should assess your body and show you which areas need to be sculpted to accomplish your objectives. The body is three-dimensional and needs to be sculpted as such. The goal is to have your body look better from all angles.

PREOPERATIVE VISIT

You should be instructed to have certain lab tests, i.e., blood work, chest x-ray, EKG. You may go to your family doctor, a hospital facility, or an independent lab. The physician you have chosen may arrange for the performance of these tests.

You may sign all of your surgical consent forms, and be given pre- and postoperative instructions at this time. You should also be given your prescriptions for before and after surgery. Make sure that everything that you and your physician have agreed on is stated on your consent form.

PRESCRIPTIONS

Some or all of these may be prescribed, in addition to others not listed.

- multvitamins—to be taken ten days to two weeks before and after surgery
- vitamin C—500 milligrams twice daily, to be taken ten days to two weeks before and after surgery
- pain medication
- antinausea medication
- oral antibiotics
- sleeping medication

Be sure to follow your doctor's instructions.

PRE- AND POSTOPERATIVE INSTRUCTIONS

These suggestions are intended to make you more comfortable and help you heal. To learn more, turn to the section on recovery in this chapter. Your doctor may have different or additional instructions. Follow them to the letter.

- Stop smoking, discontinue the use of alcohol, and stop taking vitamin E and any medications containing aspirin or ibuprofen (two weeks pre- and postoperative is usually recommended). Check with your doctor regarding any other medications (including homeopathic/herbal products) that you are currently taking.
- Know how and when to take your prescriptions.
- Know how to cleanse the surgical areas the night before or morning of your surgery.
- Do not have any food (including gum or mints) or drink (including water) for a minimum of six to eight hours prior to surgery. (Follow your surgical facility's preoperative instructions.)
- Have someone drive you to and from surgery.
- Have someone stay with you the first night after surgery (optimally, the first twenty-four hours).
- If the procedure requires a postoperative garment (to wear four to six weeks after surgery), it may be provided. You may want to purchase a second garment to wear while you launder the other.

- Some doctors supply pads to apply directly over the incisions. Others recommend that you purchase sanitary pads and/or Depends.

- Do not sunbathe or use tanning beds, especially while bruising is visible. (The pigmentation of the skin may change permanently.) Optimally, these should be avoided completely for skin care and health.

- Avoid aerobic activity for at least three weeks after surgery.

- Do not drive for at least twenty-four hours after surgery and/or while taking pain medication.

Recovery

Everyone heals differently. Healing is affected by your genetics, your physical and emotional well-being, whether you smoke and/or drink alcohol, your pain tolerance, the extent of the surgery, and how well you follow the doctor's instructions. Recovery from liposuction can take, on an average, from four days to one week.

FIRST DAY POSTOPERATIVE

You may want to sleep the first day after surgery. You could experience tenderness with movement, similar to the way you would feel if you had had an extremely strenuous workout.

SWELLING AND BRUISING

You can expect to experience some swelling and bruising after surgery. By the third week, you may still have some minor swelling, which can last for months (as long as six to nine). However, the bruising should be gone by the third week but could possibly last for six weeks.

NUMBNESS AND ITCHING

You may also have some temporary numbness, which should dissipate in a maximum of six months. If the incision sites itch, gently rub the areas—do not scratch them.

DRAINAGE FROM INCISIONS

For the first few days, there could be some drainage of the tumescent solution from the incisions (pinkish to reddish in color). It can be heavy at times—do not be alarmed. It is normal and expected. You may want to cover your bed linens with plastic and an old towel, and possibly lay an old towel on the floor beside your bed.

BODY POSITION

Elevate your legs as much as possible when sitting or lying down to help alleviate swelling of your feet and ankles. However, doctors usually recommend that you get up and start walking as soon as possible.

LOOSE-FITTING CLOTHES

Due to the swelling and drainage, plan on wearing loose-fitting, comfortable garments that you won't mind staining. Garments you do stain can usually be cleaned with peroxide and/or colorfast detergent.

WALKING/EXERCISE

By the second day, you may be allowed to start walking around the house. Many patients say that the third day is the most uncomfortable, so do not overdo it— listen to your body. If you feel tired, rest. By the fourth day, you can possibly resume your normal routine, except for strenuous activity or heavy lifting. Most physicians recommend that you wait a minimum of two to three weeks to resume aerobic exercise.

COMPRESSION GARMENTS AND DRESSINGS

Over the pads (at the incision sites), you may be required to wear a compression garment or elastic tape continuously for the first few days. After that, and for the next few weeks (according to your doctor's instructions), you should be allowed to remove the garment in order to bathe or shower. Most patients feel more comfortable with it on and choose to wear it longer than their doctor requires.

ULTRASOUND THERAPY AND MASSAGE

Many physicians recommend ultrasound therapy and massage for two to three weeks. This can aid in the healing process and help to smooth any irregularities.

SUTURES

If there are any sutures, they should be removed in about one week.

WEIGHT GAIN

Once fat cells are suctioned out with liposuction, they cannot return. However, every single fat cell is *not* removed in these areas. As a result, if there is a weight gain after liposuction, fat can still accumulate in these areas. It may be more evenly distributed and not as localized.

Pain

As with recovery times, pain tolerance is different for everyone. What one person may consider pain, another person may consider discomfort.

LEVEL OF PAIN/DISCOMFORT

Generally, with liposuction there is minimal pain during the postoperative period.

PAIN MEDICATION

Most discomfort can be controlled with pain medications you have been prescribed or Extra Strength Tylenol. You may find it necessary to take pain medication for the first day or two only.

Risks/Complications

Although problems are unlikely, you need to be aware of what can happen and what action you should take. Most risks/complications will be avoided if you make an informed decision, choose a qualified physician, and follow your physician's instructions.

BLEEDING

With the new tumescent technique, and if you have followed the doctor's instructions to the letter, bleeding is unlikely.

INFECTION

Antibiotics are given to you intravenously during the procedure, and you may be instructed to take an oral antibiotic after surgery. This should make infection unlikely.

HEMATOMA

A hematoma, a collection of blood or fluid beneath the skin, is unlikely. However, if it does occur, it can be treated by drainage with a needle or compression garment.

SEROMA

When large amounts of fat are removed, a collection of serous fluid can accumulate in the space between the skin flap and the muscle. If there is a leakage of clear yellow to blood-tinged fluid from the incision site, report it immediately to your physician. The fluid can be withdrawn with a syringe. This may occur more than once.

ASYMMETRY

Small revisions (touch-up) may be necessary.

IRREGULARITIES

Rippling, waviness, or dimpling of treated areas can occur. Some of these can be touched up; some cannot. See "Ultrasonic Assisted Liposuction (UAL)," page 218. *Note:* Most doctors will not charge for touch-ups performed in a certain time period from the original surgery. Ask your doctor what that time frame is. However, a facility fee and/or anesthesia fee will likely be charged.

HIGH-VOLUME LIPOSUCTION

Lately, a lot of media attention has been given to high-volume liposuction and its potential risks/dangers. The ideal candidate for liposuction is someone within 10 percent of her target weight. So if you are thinking of using liposuction as a weight-loss program, think again. In some cases, doctors consider the removal of over 5 pounds of fat to be a high-volume procedure. Certainly, if more fat than that is expected to be removed, the procedure will be longer, requiring an overnight stay with constant monitoring of the patient.

Potential risks include infection, fluid imbalances, shock, and blood clots. These are all potentially life-threatening complications. Do your homework before you submit to high-volume liposuction.

$\mathcal{N}$ose Reshaping–Rhinoplasty

"The concept of rhinoplasty is to refine, realign, and reposition the nasal tissues. This is accomplished by rearranging cartilage and bone to alter the shape of the nose." [1]

Rhinoplasty is commonly known as a "nose job" or nose reshaping. It is one of the top five cosmetic procedures and is performed on people of all ages. It is very rewarding because of the visual improvement and psychological satisfaction, and is quite often performed on teenagers. Rhinoplasty is the most difficult and complex cosmetic surgery procedure; more than any other cosmetic surgery, it is considered an art. Because of this, as with any surgical procedure, it is extremely important to be informed. The following section will help you. Here are some interesting facts about rhinoplasty.

- Teenagers requesting this procedure need to be assessed to determine if most of their growth spurts have occurred.

- Revisions are not uncommon—swelling during the procedure can sometimes mask imperfections. Additionally, there is no way to gauge exactly how the body will heal.

- A hump/bump can be removed or the nose can be made smaller, narrower, or shorter but not always wider or larger.

- Cartilage implants are sometimes necessary—cartilage may be removed from one part of the nose (the septum) and grafted to another (usually the tip); cartilage or bone from ear, skull, or rib may also be used. If adequate cartilage is not available, a synthetic material, e.g., Gore-Tex, may be used.

---

[1] Diana Barry, *Nips & Tucks,* (Santa Monica, Calif.: General Publishing Group, 1996).

- It is not unusual to have a chin augmentation (mentoplasty) or chin reduction in conjunction with a rhinoplasty to bring the profile into balance.

- If breathing is obstructed, the septum can be repaired at the same time (septoplasty).

Procedure

You must make some important decisions if you choose this procedure—the location of the incisions (technique) and your desired look. Educate yourself so that you can be a part of this decision-making process. The surgical options you choose may be determining factors in your physician selection. Remember that different doctors use different techniques and usually recommend the one(s) in which they are trained and experienced. In general, if you undergo a rhinoplasty, here's what you can expect.

ANESTHESIA

Rhinoplasty can be performed under intravenous sedation with local anesthesia or under general anesthesia. The type of anesthesia is dependent on the extent of the procedure to be performed, the doctor's choice, and the patient's medical history or desires.

TECHNIQUES

Two techniques are currently being used. The technique your surgeon uses may depend on his training and experience.

Traditional—"Closed"

All of the incisions are made inside the nostrils.

Newer—"Open"

An incision is made on the columella, the central portion below the tip of the nose between the nostrils (open rhinoplasty). This technique can take a little longer, but it allows the surgeon a better view and greater access to the inner structures. If a reduction in the size of the nostrils is desired, the incisions can be made in the crease where the side of the nostril meets the upper lip and cheek (alar incision). The incisions usually heal to a very fine, inconspicuous scar.

STEPS IN THE NOSE RESHAPING PROCEDURE

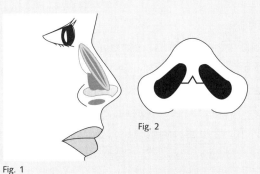

Fig. 1

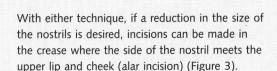

Fig. 2

Traditional "Closed" Procedure
All of the incisions are made inside the nostrils (Figure 1).

Newer "Open" Procedure
An incision is made on the columella, which is the central portion below the tip of the nose, between the nostrils (Figure 2).

With either technique, if a reduction in the size of the nostrils is desired, incisions can be made in the crease where the side of the nostril meets the upper lip and cheek (alar incision) (Figure 3).

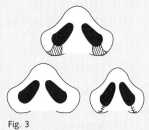

Fig. 3

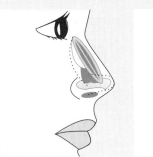

Fig. 4

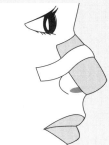

Fig. 5

The skin is separated from the underlying bone and cartilage, and the surgeon works to reshape the structures by incising, filing, trimming, repositioning, and sculpting the cartilage and nasal bones (Figure 4).

Very small stitches are placed to close the incision(s), and a splint is applied to protect the nose (Figure 5).

Whichever technique is used, once anesthesia has been administered, the nose is further anesthetized with a local anesthetic that helps shrink the mucous membranes and control bleeding. The skin is separated from the underlying bone and cartilage, and the surgeon works to reshape the structures by incising, filing, trimming, repositioning, and sculpting the cartilage and nasal bones. Contrary to popular belief, the nose is not broken during the operation. Medical-grade chisels (osteotomes) are used to create small cuts in the nasal bones, making the bones moldable if the desired result is a narrower, straighter, or refined shape.

SUTURES AND DRESSINGS

Very small stitches are placed to close the incision(s), and a splint is applied to protect the nose. Your doctor should remove this in about a week. A drip pad is placed under the nose to catch any oozing blood (you can change this pad as needed). Additionally, packing may or may not be inserted into the nostrils and, if used, is removed by the doctor or nurse in three to five days. Today, packing is used less often. However, there may be indications for its use in certain cases.

LENGTH OF SURGICAL PROCEDURE

Rhinoplasty can take from one and one-half to four hours, depending on the extent of the surgery to be done. The time can be increased if the procedure is a revision or a reconstructive procedure.

Prior to Surgery

Before surgery, you and your doctor will first make several important decisions. Then you will prepare for surgery and be given prescriptions and instructions. The following sections will give you an overview of the process.

ASSESSMENT

Bring magazine pictures of noses that you like to your initial consultation with your doctor—but remember, your new nose has to fit the shape and size of your face. This procedure requires an in-depth evaluation of your nose, facial structure, and skin type. Your height and bone structure are also considered. As a result of this assessment, the doctor may make a computer image (or sketch) of the nose that you have agreed upon.

It is imperative that you understand there are no guarantees that your nose can be made to exactly duplicate a computer image or picture. This is a complex and delicate operation. The surgeon cannot judge how your body will respond in the healing process. Be absolutely clear and in agreement with your doctor about how you want your new nose to look. The doctor should devise a plan to achieve results that will not only improve the shape of your nose but also the appearance of your entire face.

At this time, the decision to have a chin augmentation (mentoplasty) or chin reduction in conjunction with a rhinoplasty will be made. Any breathing problem will be assessed, and your doctor may recommend a septoplasty (straightening of the septum), which can be done at the same time.

PREOPERATIVE VISIT

You should be instructed to have certain lab tests, i.e., blood work, chest x-ray, EKG. You may go to your family doctor, a hospital facility, or an independent lab. The physician you have chosen may arrange for the performance of these tests.

You may sign all of your surgical consent forms and be given pre- and postoperative instructions at this time. You should also be given your prescriptions for before and after surgery. Make sure that everything you and your physician have agreed on is stated on your consent form.

PRESCRIPTIONS

Some or all of these may be prescribed, in addition to others not listed.

- multivitamins—to be taken ten days to two weeks before and after surgery
- vitamin C—500 milligrams twice daily, to be taken ten days to two weeks before and after surgery
- pain medication
- anti-inflammatory medication (some physicians require this before and after surgery to reduce swelling and bruising)
- antinausea medication
- oral antibiotics
- sleeping medication

Be sure to follow your doctor's instructions.

PRE- AND POSTOPERATIVE INSTRUCTIONS

These suggestions are intended to make you more comfortable and help you heal. To learn more, turn to the section on recovery in this chapter. Your doctor may have different or additional instructions. Follow them to the letter.

- Stop smoking, discontinue the use of alcohol, and stop taking vitamin E and any medications containing aspirin or ibuprofen (two weeks pre- and post-operative is usually recommended). Check with your doctor regarding any other medications (including homeopathic/herbal products) that you are currently taking.

- Eliminate milk products from your diet a few days before surgery and during the initial healing period (milk products produce mucus).

- Be sure you understand how and when to take/apply your prescriptions.

- Know how to cleanse the surgical areas the night before or the morning of your surgery.

- Do not have any food (includes gum or mints) or drink (including water) for a minimum of six to eight hours prior to surgery. (Follow your surgical facility's preoperative instructions.)

- Have someone drive you to and from surgery.

- Have someone stay with you the first night after surgery (the first twenty-four hours, optimally).

- If the procedure requires a splint, this may be applied by the doctor or nurse immediately after the procedure. This must be kept dry.

- Change the drip pad (two-inch by two-inch gauze) as needed.

- Do not sunbathe or use tanning beds at least two weeks prior to surgery. (For optimal skin care and health, these should be avoided completely.) After surgery, you must protect your nose from the sun for at least six weeks. The longer, the better.

- Avoid aerobic activity for a minimum of three to four weeks after surgery. You do not want to do anything that could elevate your blood pressure or cause your nose to bleed.

- Avoid contact sports for six weeks.

- Avoid diving for two months.

- Do not drive for at least twenty-four hours after surgery and/or while taking pain medication.

- Do not wear glasses for the first two months unless okayed by your doctor (and then they must be taped to your forehead). Or wear contact lenses. Some glasses are heavy and could cause a groove at the bridge or place unnecessary pressure on the new structure.

- Lift nothing heavier than a small telephone book.

- Do not blow your nose until instructed. When instructed, blow using alternating nostrils so that pressure is not built up.

- Sneeze with your mouth open to minimize pressure.

- You may want to keep some type of lip balm or petroleum jelly on your lips—otherwise they may become dry because you will be breathing through your mouth.

- You may find that your nose and/or surrounding skin are oilier than normal. This could last for several weeks.

- Most doctors instruct that cold compresses are to be applied for twenty minutes every hour for a minimum of forty-eight hours.

- Consider sleeping alone for the first week or so in an effort to protect against accidental blows to the nose while sleeping.

- Rest and relax for the first week.

- Do not apply makeup until your doctor instructs you.

- Take special care not to injure the nose in any way during the first six weeks.

Recovery

Everyone heals differently. Healing is affected by your genetics, physical and emotional well-being, whether you smoke and/or drink alcohol, your pain tolerance, the extent of the surgery, and how well you follow the doctor's instructions. Plan on approximately seven days for the initial healing period.

POSTOPERATIVE PHYSICIAN APPOINTMENTS

Your doctor may want to see you the day after surgery. That activity alone may be all you will want to do, or should do, that day. After your appointment, go home and rest. If there is packing, it is usually removed by the doctor or nurse in one to three days. Your sutures (if external) are removed in about a week, along with the splint. Do not expect to see a perfectly shaped nose when the splint is removed. Your nose may possibly appear "turned up" and the tip swollen from the effects of the dressing and swelling. You will probably have appointments to return to the doctor's office in about two weeks, and then again in six weeks.

FIRST DAY POSTOPERATIVE

You will probably want to sleep the first day after surgery. Your nose will be stuffy, your mouth will be dry, and you could be swollen and bruised around the central portion of your face, including the eyes.

STUFFINESS

Your nose will be stuffy for approximately two to three weeks. Breathing through your mouth will make your mouth and lips dry.

SWELLING AND BRUISING

The swelling in the central portion of your face should lessen in the first few days, with some minor swelling remaining in the first weeks. However, it can take up to a year or longer for all of the swelling to disappear (especially for the tip). This swelling, if noticeable at all, may only be noticeable to you. During that time it can come and go, as it can be affected by fluid retention caused by the menstrual cycle or the consumption of salty or spicy foods. You can expect to be black and blue in the central portion of your face. This can last on the average anywhere from five days to several weeks, but it will diminish daily. Remember—everyone is different. You will probably notice that the bruising drops (travels lower in the face) over the first few days. This is normal. You can apply makeup (regular and/or camouflage) after the sutures and/or splint are removed.

DRESSINGS

A number of dressings are used in a rhinoplasty. Your physician will give you specific instructions.

Drip Pad

Change your drip pad (two-inch by two-inch gauze under your nose), as needed, to catch any light bloody discharge. For the first few hours after surgery, this may mean several times an hour. The discharge should progressively diminish and should stop by the next morning. A small amount of bloody discharge from the nose is normal. However, if your nose starts bleeding, contact your doctor immediately.

Splint

Your physician will have applied a splint to protect the nose. Do not get it wet—be careful when bathing. Your doctor or nurse will usually remove this at the same time as the sutures—in about a week. Makeup (regular and/or camouflage) can be applied after the sutures and/or splint are removed.

Packing

Packing may or may not be inserted into the nostrils and will be removed by the doctor or nurse in one to three days. Today, packing is generally used less often. However, there may be indications for its use in certain cases.

COLD COMPRESSES

Cold compresses may relieve some of the discomfort and can greatly reduce the swelling. These should be applied every hour for twenty minutes for a minimum of forty-eight hours (some doctors recommend seventy-two hours) after surgery. Ice should never be placed directly on the skin. Either use cold compresses or place a cloth between the ice bag and your skin. In some cases, your doctor may have instructed you *not* to use cold compresses. Follow your doctor's instructions.

BODY POSITION

It is imperative that you keep your head elevated at all times for at least the first week, optimally two weeks. Surround yourself with pillows or sleep on a recliner. Under no circumstances should you lie face down or bend over for a minimum of one to two weeks. If you need to pick something up, squat with your knees bent. Do not pick up anything heavier than a small telephone book.

WALKING/EXERCISE

By the third day, you may be allowed to start walking around the house. Do not overdo it—listen to your body. If you feel tired, rest. By the end of the first week, you can possibly resume some of your normal routine, except for strenuous activity or heavy lifting. Most physicians recommend that you wait a minimum of three to four weeks to resume aerobic exercise.

INCISION LINES

Your scars (if external) may remain red for four to six weeks and should gradually fade. Most scars become barely noticeable over time.

CARE OF THE NOSE

It is extremely important that the nose is not injured in any way for the first two months. Immediately after surgery, if you must blow your nose, alternate nostrils so that pressure is not built up. Also, if you must sneeze, do so with your mouth open. Avoid wearing your glasses/sunglasses, or tape them to your forehead as instructed by your doctor. Or wear contact lenses. Do not rub the nose for six months after surgery. Additionally, with a rhinoplasty, the skin on the nose is more susceptible to sun damage and frostbite. For the first year after surgery, when you are outside during the day, wear sunblock. Also, in the winter, cover your nose with a scarf.

Pain

As with recovery times, pain tolerance is different for everyone. What one person may consider pain, another person may consider discomfort.

LEVEL OF PAIN/DISCOMFORT

Generally, with rhinoplasty there can be minimal to moderate discomfort. Some people experience absolutely no discomfort at all.

PAIN MEDICATION

Most discomfort can be controlled with pain medications you have been prescribed or Extra Strength Tylenol. You may find it necessary to take pain medication for the first day or two only.

Risks/Complications

Although problems are unlikely, you need to be aware of what can happen and what action you should take. Most risks/complications will be avoided if you make an informed decision, choose a qualified physician, and follow your physician's instructions.

BLEEDING

Call your doctor immediately.

INFECTION

Continue taking antibiotics as instructed, and do not put anything up the nose.

BREATHING PROBLEMS

Breathing problems are unlikely.

COSMETIC DEFORMITIES

Problems may include a hump, a bump, asymmetry, collapse, or arching nostrils. The need or desire for revision is not unusual.

Soft Tissue Fillers

Soft tissue fillers are substances that are injected or implanted to make a body part fuller, or to fill out lines, wrinkles, and creases.

Many patients choose soft tissue fillers to help turn back the hands of time, either as a procedure by itself or in conjunction with surgical facial procedures. As an example, a patient may have very deep nasolabial folds (creases that run from beside the nostrils to the sides of the mouth). A face-lift minimally addresses these folds, so that it may be necessary to fill them with soft tissue fillers. Here are some important facts about soft tissue fillers.

- Everyone reacts differently to the introduction of foreign materials into the body.
- The effect of some soft tissue injectable fillers is temporary.
- Fillers can be inserted in conjunction with other facial surgeries, peels, and/or liposuction.
- Soft tissue fillers usually require local anesthesia only.
- Fillers can be a preliminary step to postpone more complex procedures, such as a face-lift.

Procedure

A number of different types of tissue filler materials are available. You and your physician must take into consideration your desired look and whether you are comfortable with a temporary or possibly permanent solution. Remember that different doctors use different techniques and materials and usually recommend the one(s) in which they are trained and experienced. All of these factors may be determine your physician selection. Most physicians perform these procedures in their offices versus a surgical facility.

TECHNIQUES

The following sections will give you an overview of some of the most common soft tissue fillers being used by physicians.

Collagen

Collagen, which is derived from cows, is effective on fine and deep lines, contour deformities, and some types of scars, including acne scars. It is also used for lip augmentation. However, it is not approved for any other part of the body except the face.

The different types of collagen are as follows. Which type you choose will be determined by what you want to accomplish.

Zyderm—lighter form used for superficial lines; usually requires multiple treatments.

Zyplast—used for deeper lines; usually requires only one treatment.

Allergic reactions can occur, so it is necessary to undergo a skin test (usually on the underside of the arm) thirty days prior to collagen injections to determine any sensitivity or allergy. Even with a negative test result, there can still be an allergic reaction that can develop immediately, or over time. Collagen should not be injected into anyone with a connective tissue disease (e.g., lupus, scleroderma).

Collagen is injected via a syringe, and does not usually require any type of anesthesia. Mild discomfort may be experienced during the injections and there may be some swelling, bruising, and numbness at the sites for the first two days. However, cold compresses can be applied to relieve any discomfort and swelling. Any bruising can be covered up with makeup immediately after treatment.

The disadvantages of collagen include the following:

- Repeated injections are necessary to maintain results.
- The more it is done, the greater the risk of scar tissue formation.
- There is the suspicion that bovine collagen may play a role in the development of autoimmune diseases. However, there is no current research data to confirm this.

The effects are temporary; they can last anywhere from a few weeks to a year (average is two to six months). Some physicians believe that the more immobile the treated area is kept, the longer the collagen will last.

Fat Transfer—The Body's Own Fat (Autologous)

Autologous fat is effective on deep lines (such as the nasolabial folds) and when used to plump up areas such as the lips. It cannot be used on the hands or the breasts. There is little possibility of rejection, because the fat is from the patient's own body.

Fat transfer can be performed under local anesthesia with oral analgesics and sedatives, local anesthesia with intravenous sedation, or with general anesthesia. The type of anesthesia is dependent on the extent of procedures to be performed, the doctor's choice, and the patient's medical history or desires. Fat is harvested from a donor site (usually buttocks or abdomen). If liposuction or a blepharoplasty (eyelids) is being performed at the same time, fat from those sites can be utilized. Blood and antiseptic solution are separated from the harvested fat (the fat must be treated very gently so that the cell structure is not disturbed). The fat is then placed very gently in its new location through a tiny incision. A stitch or two may be placed at the donor and graft sites, if required. The procedure can take approximately thirty to ninety minutes, depending on the extent of the areas to be treated.

Some swelling, bruising, and numbness may be experienced at the sites for the first two days, along with mild discomfort. Cold compresses can be applied to relieve any discomfort and swelling. Any bruising can be covered up with makeup in a few days, according to your doctor's instructions.

The effects may or may not be permanent. Some physicians believe that the more immobile the treated area is kept, the longer the fat transfer will last.

Note: Harvested fat can be stored under refrigerated conditions for future use. However, there are differing opinions as to the maximum amount of time it can be stored, and why it would be necessary to do so, since harvesting more fat is a simple procedure.

Fat Grafting—Dermal Grafts

Dermal grafts are used for filling deep depressions, such as the nasolabial folds. They can also be placed along the vermilion border (edge of the lips) to create an enhanced appearance and may be used in conjunction with other procedures (dermabrasion, laser resurfacing) to eliminate acne scars.

The different types of dermal grafts are as follows.

Autologous—derived from the patient's body; also known as autologous fat grafts.

AlloDerm—derived from sanitized cadaver skin.

Human collagen—from donor other than the patient.

Allergic reactions rarely occur because a dermal graft is not a foreign substance. If derived from the patient's own body, a piece of skin is harvested, usually from the buttocks or groin, and the incision is then sutured. Otherwise, it is supplied to your physician through a medical supply company. The dermis is separated from the epidermis and shaped. An incision is placed at the wrinkle or depression to be filled in, and the graft is inserted. This incision is then sutured.

Some swelling may be experienced at the graft site for about two days. At the graft and donor sites, there may be some bruising and numbness, which may last for a few weeks. Cold compresses can be applied to relieve any discomfort and swelling, according to your physician's instructions. The graft becomes incorporated with the surrounding tissues and cannot be removed after two to four weeks. If an infection occurs, the patient is treated with antibiotics.

The effects may or may not be permanent. Some physicians believe that the more immobile the treated area is kept, the longer the fat graft will last.

Synthetic Materials

A number of synthetic materials are currently being used as soft tissue fillers. They are made of materials that have been used for many years as prostheses and/or for grafting and are effective for deep creases such as the nasolabial folds or furrows between the brows. They can also be placed along the vermilion border (edge of the lips) to create an enhanced appearance. A major advantage of synthetic materials is that they are easy to revise and/or remove. If misplacement occurs, a revision is easily done.

Some available synthetic products are as follows:

- *GORE Subcutaneous Augmentation Material (S.A.M.)* made by Gore (Gore-Tex) is pliable and microporous (tissue can grow into it).

- *SoftForm* made by Collagen, Inc., is a hollow material (tissue can grow into it).

- *Medpor* is a porous textured polyethylene, which allows vessels to incorporate into it.

Minimal cases of allergic reactions have been reported. If the material is placed too close to the surface of the skin, the material may extrude (expel or protrude). A revision procedure would be required.

A tiny incision is placed at each end of the area to be treated. The synthetic material is placed under the skin with a small tube, and one suture is placed at each incision. Some swelling, bruising, and numbness at the sites may be experienced for the first two days. Cold compresses can be applied to relieve any discomfort and swelling. Any bruising can be covered up with makeup in a few days, according to your doctor's instructions. If an infection occurs, the patient is treated with antibiotics. The effects may be permanent.

Research is ongoing to develop the perfect soft tissue filler that is natural-feeling, safe, and permanent. New and/or improved soft tissue filler products are being introduced every year. As with any surgical procedure, it is important to be informed. Make sure that everything you and your physician have agreed on is stated on your consent form, such as the material he will be using.

Tummy Tuck–Abdominoplasty

This procedure is a way of tightening the abdominal muscles, and/or removing excess fatty tissue and sagging skin from the middle and lower abdomen.

Many abdominoplasty patients are women whose abdominal muscles have been overstretched and have not returned to normal after one or more pregnancies. In older candidates, a significant weight loss may have resulted in sagging skin (loss of elasticity). With any surgical procedure, it is important to be informed. However, because of the significant scar that abdominoplasty produces, it is even more important for you to educate yourself. The following section will help you. Here are some important facts about abdominoplasty.

- Liposuction on the flank and hip areas may be performed in conjunction with a tummy tuck to achieve a better contour.
- This procedure is not recommended for smokers.

Procedure

Abdominoplasty does produce a noticeable scar. However, if the skin has lost its elasticity, liposuction of the abdomen will not be sufficient; loose skin will remain. Some patients are willing to trade a firm abdomen for a scar. Remember that different doctors use different techniques and usually recommend the one(s) in which they are trained and experienced. You and your physician must take into consideration your desired look. In general, if you do make the decision to undergo an abdominoplasty, here's what you can expect.

ANESTHESIA

An abdominoplasty may be performed under general anesthesia or spinal anesthesia. However, the type of anesthesia used is dependent on the procedure to be performed, the doctor's choice, and the patient's medical history or desires.

OPTIONS

A number of different options are available for the abdominal area depending on the elasticity of your skin and laxity (relaxation) of your abdominal muscles. Your physician will recommend the procedure he feels will best accomplish your desired look.

Liposuction

This may be recommended if there is just excess fat and the skin has not lost its ability to shrink back (elasticity) or redrape. (See "Liposuction," page 217.)

Endoscopic Abdominoplasty

This technique may be recommended if the only concern is the laxity of the abdominal muscle, and there is minimal skin and/or fatty tissue. Tiny incisions are made in the navel and just above the pubic bone, and the abdominal muscles are pulled together and sutured.

Mini- or Partial Abdominoplasty

Bulging of the lower abdomen only (below the navel) is corrected. The candidates for this procedure are usually thin and have sagging skin and very little fat. The incision is made just above the pubis and is smaller than that of a complete abdominoplasty. The skin is separated from the underlying tissue and lifted up to the umbilicus (navel). The excess skin is removed and the abdominal muscles are tightened, if necessary. The skin is then sutured into place. A drain may or may not be placed. Recovery time may be shorter than that of a complete abdominoplasty because it is less invasive.

Complete Abdominoplasty

This may be recommended to remove excess fatty tissue and skin above and below the navel, as well as to tighten the abdominal muscles. An incision is usually made from hip to hip across the lower abdomen as well as an incision around the umbilicus. The skin is separated from the underlying tissue and lifted all the way up to the rib cage. The navel is left attached to the underlying abdominal tissue.

If there are deep layers of fatty tissue, some may be removed by cutting them away from the skin, or liposuction may be performed. Liposuction may also be used at this time to contour the hip and flank areas. The abdominal muscles are then pulled together and sutured. The resected skin is then pulled down very tightly, and the excess skin below the navel is removed. The surgeon repositions the navel and sutures it into place. The incisions are then closed either with staples or sutures.

STEPS IN THE TUMMY TUCK PROCEDURE

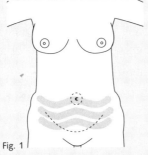

Fig. 1

The incision usually spans from hip to hip across the lower abdomen, as well as an incision around the umbilicus (navel) (Figure 1).

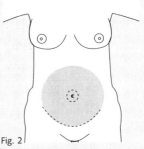

Fig. 2

The skin is separated from the underlying tissue and lifted all the way up to the rib cage. The navel is left attached to the underlying abdominal tissue (Figure 2).

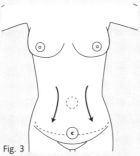

Fig. 3

Deep layers of fatty tissue may be removed by cutting them away from the skin, and/or liposuction may be performed. The abdominal muscles are pulled together and sutured (Figure 3).

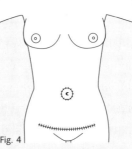

Fig. 4

The resected skin is pulled down very tightly, and the excess skin below the navel is removed. The navel is repositioned and sutured into place. Incisions are closed either with staples or sutures. Drains may be placed (Figure 4).

DRAINS

A complete abdominoplasty, and possibly a mini-abdominoplasty, may require drains that are sutured into place. A catheter may also be placed.

DRESSINGS

For all abdominal options, dressings are applied to the incisions and while you are still in the operating room, an abdominal support garment is generally applied.

LENGTH OF SURGICAL PROCEDURE

A complete abdominoplasty should take from two to five hours. Most physicians require an overnight stay in the hospital or surgical facility because respiration needs to be monitored and the general anesthesia may cause nausea. The nausea must be controlled for the first twenty-four hours because vomiting could tear the repaired muscles.

Prior to Surgery

Before surgery, you and your doctor will first make several important decisions. Then you will prepare for surgery and be given prescriptions and instructions. The following will give you an overview of the process.

ASSESSMENT

Your physician should evaluate and assess the location of the fat in the abdomen, along with the laxity of the skin and abdominal muscle. Your doctor may recommend the endoscopic approach, a mini-abdominoplasty, complete abdominoplasty, and/or liposuction. Liposuction may be performed in the hip and flank areas in conjunction with the abdominoplasty to contour the area. It is critical to have a thorough assessment. Be absolutely clear and in agreement with your doctor about your desired look.

Note: Many doctors choose not to perform an abdominoplasty on smokers. Smoking diminishes blood flow and may result in the abdominal skin not surviving the surgery. Scars would replace this dead tissue, potentially causing severe disfigurement.

LOCATION OF INCISIONS

Discuss with your physician the location of the incisions. You may want to bring your bathing suit to your consultation. Put it on to show your physician its lines so that the location of the incisions can be planned. Also, take into consideration the type of undergarments you wear. If the location of the incisions is a major concern for you, you may even want to bring your bathing suit the day of surgery. In that way, your physician can mark the location of the incision with the suit as a guide. Your doctor may attempt to accommodate your choice for the location of the incisions, but this is no guarantee that the scars will not be visible once healing has taken place.

PREOPERATIVE VISIT

You should be instructed to have certain lab tests, i.e., blood work, chest x-ray, EKG. For the lab tests, you may go to your family doctor, an independent lab, or a hospital facility. The physician you have chosen may arrange for the performance of these tests.

You may sign all of your surgical consent forms and be given pre- and postoperative instructions at this time. You should also be given your prescriptions for before and after surgery. Make sure that everything you and your physician have agreed on is stated on your consent form.

PRESCRIPTIONS

Some or all of these may be prescribed, in addition to others not listed.

- multivitamins—to be taken ten days to two weeks before and after surgery
- vitamin C—500 milligrams twice daily, to be taken ten days to two weeks before and after surgery
- pain medication
- antinausea medication
- oral antibiotics and/or ointment
- sleeping medication
- steroids (i.e. cortisone), to minimize swelling

Be sure to follow your doctor's instructions.

PRE- AND POSTOPERATIVE INSTRUCTIONS

These suggestions are intended to make you more comfortable and help you heal. To learn more, turn to the section on recovery in this chapter. Your doctor may have different or additional instructions. Follow them to the letter.

- Stop smoking (see note, page 248), discontinue the use of alcohol, and stop taking vitamin E and any medications containing aspirin or ibuprofen (two weeks pre- and postoperative is usually recommended). Check with your doctor regarding any other medications (including homeopathic/herbal products) that you are currently taking.

- Be sure you understand how and when to take/apply your prescriptions.

- Know how to cleanse the surgical areas the night before or morning of your surgery.

- Do not have any food (including gum or mints) or drink (including water) for a minimum of six to eight hours prior to surgery. (Follow your surgical facility's preoperative instructions.)

- Have someone drive you to and from surgery (probably the day after surgery).

- Have someone stay with you the first night after surgery (the first twenty-four to forty-eight hours preferably). Most physicians require an overnight stay in the hospital or surgical facility.

- Dressings and/or drains, if required, should be applied by the doctor or nurse immediately after the procedure. Your physician will instruct you as to the amount of time an abdominal binder is to be worn—usually between four and six weeks.

- Purchase a second garment so that you always have a clean one.

- Follow directions regarding any ointments to be applied and/or cleansing of incisions.

- Do not sunbathe or use tanning beds at least two weeks prior to surgery. (For optimal skin care and health, these activities should be avoided completely.) After surgery, avoid the sun unless your abdomen is protected.

- Avoid aerobic activity for at least four to six weeks after surgery.

- Most physicians recommend that you get up and start taking short walks around the house by the second day, increasing the amount each day.

- Avoid exercise that directly affects the abdominal muscles for two to three months.

- Try not to drive or ride in a car for ten to fourteen days. You must avoid accidents to give the deep tissues adequate time to heal.

- For the first week to two weeks, when lying down, lie on your back, keeping your head and knees elevated (jackknife position). Place pillows to support your head and upper back and prop up your knees with pillows. A recliner works perfectly.

- When you are up and walking, at first you will need to bend over at the waist to prevent tension at the suture line. You will be able to straighten up gradually as the skin on your abdomen stretches.

- Lift nothing heavier than a small telephone book.

- Do not rub your skin. Be extremely gentle for a minimum of a month.

- Expect numbness in the areas treated for eight to twelve weeks.

- Your doctor may instruct you to apply cold compresses, usually twenty minutes every hour for a minimum of forty-eight hours.

- Rest and relax for the first week.

- As your incisions start to heal, they may itch. Do not scratch them. Ask your doctor if you can apply cream or ointment to relieve the itching, and only use what is recommended.

Recovery

Everyone heals differently. Healing is affected by your genetics, your physical and emotional well-being, whether you smoke and/or drink alcohol, your pain tolerance, the extent of the surgery, and how well you follow the doctor's instructions. Plan on approximately two to three weeks for the initial healing period.

PHYSICIAN'S INSTRUCTIONS

With all surgical procedures, it is always important to follow your doctor's instructions. *It is absolutely imperative that instructions are followed to the letter with an abdominoplasty.* This is a major operation.

POSTOPERATIVE PHYSICIAN APPOINTMENTS

In approximately five days, you should have your first postoperative appointment. If drains were inserted (and not removed during the first twenty-four to forty-eight hours), they may be removed at this time. Your next appointment may be on the twelfth to fourteenth day after surgery. Your sutures may or may not be removed at this time, depending on how well the incisions are healing. You should schedule an appointment to return to the doctor's office at about three weeks after surgery and then again in approximately six weeks, three months, and six months.

FIRST DAY POSTOPERATIVE

Many physicians require an overnight stay in the hospital or surgical facility because respiration needs to be monitored, and the general anesthesia may cause nausea. Nausea needs to be controlled for the first twenty-four hours because vomiting could tear the repaired muscles.

You may want to sleep the first day after surgery. The abdominal area may feel sore and very tight, and you may experience swelling and bruising. Expect a level of numbness and a tight feeling in the treated areas. You will need help getting in and out of bed for the first few days.

SWELLING AND BRUISING

The swelling should lessen daily, with some minor swelling remaining after the first few weeks. If there is increased swelling and/or bruising and tenderness, this may represent a hematoma (collection of blood) under the skin. Contact your physician immediately for evaluation. The bruising may last, on the average, anywhere from five days to several weeks but should diminish daily. Remember—everyone heals differently.

NUMBNESS AND ITCHING

You may also have some temporary numbness, which should dissipate in a maximum of six months. It can, however, last up to a year. Also, if the incision sites itch, gently rub the areas—do not scratch them. Ask your doctor if you can apply some cream or ointment to relieve the itching, and use only what is recommended.

COMPRESSION GARMENT

The physician or nurse may place an abdominal compression garment on you while you are still in the operating room. It helps reduce fluid buildup and supports and molds the skin. Most physicians require that this be worn twenty-four hours a day for four to six weeks. It should only be removed when you shower.

COLD COMPRESSES

Cold compresses applied to the abdomen may relieve some of the discomfort and can greatly reduce the swelling. These should be applied every hour for twenty minutes for a minimum of forty-eight hours (some doctors recommend seventy-two hours) after surgery. Ice should never be placed directly on the skin. Either use cold compresses or place a cloth between the ice bag and your skin. In some cases, your doctor may have instructed you *not* to use cold compresses. Follow your doctor's instructions.

BODY POSITION

It is important to keep your head and upper body elevated, with your knees propped up (jackknife position) at all times when lying down for at least the first week. Sleep on a recliner or prop yourself up with pillows. Do not lie face down for the first three weeks. Additionally, if you need to pick something up, squat with your knees bent. Do not pick up anything heavier than a small telephone book.

WALKING/EXERCISE

By the second day, you will probably be allowed to start taking short walks inside your house. However, when you are up and walking, bend at the waist to prevent tension at the suture line. You will be able to straighten up gradually as the skin on your abdomen stretches. Do not overdo it—listen to your body. If you feel tired, rest. After the first week, you can possibly resume some of your normal routine, except for strenuous activity or heavy lifting. Most physicians recommend that you wait a minimum of three to four weeks to resume aerobic exercise and two to three months for any type of abdominal exercise.

DRAINS

If drains were inserted, they may be removed during the first twenty-four to forty-eight hours or at your next physician's appointment in approximately five days. There may be some discomfort when they are removed, so you may choose to take your pain medication prior to your appointment. After that appointment, go home and rest.

BATHING

You may be given permission to shower on the third day. However, do not take tub baths until instructed by your physician.

INCISION LINES

Your sutures/staples may or may not be removed during your twelve- to fourteen-day postoperative appointment, depending on how well you are healing. Your scar may remain red for four to six weeks. It may be wider than most scars because there is a lot of tension on the incision site due to its location. However, if the scar becomes raised or thickened as well as red, then notify your physician immediately. This may represent hypertrophic scarring, which can be treated if caught early.

Pain

As with recovery times, pain tolerance is different for everyone. What one person may consider pain, another person may consider discomfort.

LEVEL OF PAIN/DISCOMFORT

Generally, with an abdominoplasty there is moderate to severe discomfort during the postoperative period. Some patients describe the discomfort as a burning sensation, which results from the muscle repair. This usually subsides in a few days.

PAIN MEDICATION

Most discomfort can be controlled with pain medications you have been prescribed. You may find it necessary to take pain medication for the first day or two only.

Risks/Complications

Although problems are unlikely, you need to be aware of what can happen and what action you should take. Most risks/complications will be avoided if you make an informed decision, choose a qualified physician, and follow your physician's instructions.

INFECTION

If there is any serious pain, heavy oozing, or fever, this should be reported immediately to the doctor. An infection can be treated with antibiotic ointments and/or oral antibiotics.

HEMATOMA

A hematoma, a collection of blood or fluid beneath the skin, is unlikely. However, if it does occur, it can be treated by drainage with a needle or with compression.

HYPERTROPHIC SCARRING

Report any signs of hypertrophic scarring immediately to your doctor; this scarring can be treated if caught early. (See "Definitions of Scarring/Skin Changes," page 56.)

SEROMA

When large amounts of fat are removed, a collection of serous fluid can accumulate in the space between the skin flap and muscle. If there is a leakage of clear yellow to blood-tinged fluid from the incision site, report it immediately to your physician. The fluid can be withdrawn with a syringe. This may occur more than once.

*V*ein Therapy

Sclerotherapy and laser light therapy are the procedures used to remove or eliminate varicose and spider veins.

Many people feel self-conscious about spider or varicose veins on their legs. Currently, the two techniques most widely used can be performed in your physician's office. One is performed via injections and the other is a totally noninvasive laser light therapy. As with any procedure, it is important to be informed.

Procedure

In the past, the only way to eliminate varicose veins was to have them removed surgically. Sclerotherapy was then introduced and has been effective in eliminating varicose veins. In the last few years, laser light therapy has been gaining in popularity. Up until recently, laser light therapy was only used in the treatment of spider veins. However, many physicians and vein therapists have recently seen good results for varicose veins. Remember that different doctors use different techniques and usually recommend the one(s) in which they are trained and experienced. All of these factors may be determine your physician selection. The following sections will give you an overview of the two most widely used techniques.

SALINE OR CHEMICAL SOLUTION INJECTIONS

Saline or chemical solutions are known as "sclerosing agents." These solution injections are used to eliminate leg veins. The injection inflames the vein, causing it to collapse. The walls of the collapsed vein then grow together so that the vein is closed. The needles used are tiny so there is minimal discomfort, if any, during the injections (slight to moderate burning). The muscles may cramp during the procedure, but cramping usually subsides in a few minutes.

Side Effects

- Some bruising may occur, which may last about one week.

- There may be some discoloration within the vein (light brown streaks), which should gradually fade. Fading may take weeks or months.

- There may be a mild itching for one to two days along the route of the vein.

- A small percentage of patients experience sloughing—a small ulceration (blister) at the injection site. This condition usually resolves with time.

- Allergic reaction to the sclerosing agent is rare, but is greater if a solution other than saline or saline with dextrose is used.

- If cramping occurs, walking will usually help.

After Treatment

Here is what you can expect following saline or chemical solution injections.

- An ointment may be applied along with a pressure bandage.

- It may be necessary to wear compression stockings for two to three weeks for varicose veins, a few days for spider veins.

- You may experience mild to moderate discomfort at the injection sites.

- Vein routes may be tender after treatment, with an uncomfortable sensation that may last one to seven days.

- Patients are encouraged to walk at least thirty minutes each day for two weeks.

- Avoid heavy exercise for one to two days.

- Avoid direct exposure to the sun for two weeks, and use sunscreen for at least six weeks (exposure to the sun or tanning beds can increase the possibility of hyperpigmentation).

More than one treatment is usually necessary to achieve the desired result.

LASER LIGHT THERAPY
(CANDELA SCLEROPLUS, PHOTODERM, ALEXANDRITE)

This noninvasive procedure can be used on varicose veins and spider veins on the legs and face. A hand-held treatment unit, which generates intense pulsed light, is held just above the surface of the skin. It is aimed at each portion of the vein to be eliminated. The treatment may feel like a pinch or the snap of a rubber band against the skin. Varicose and spider veins fade, and then slowly disappear. Local anesthesia or pain medication is usually not required.

After Treatment

Here is what you can expect following laser light therapy.

- A slight reddening of the skin and localized swelling may occur, which may last for a few days.

- Blistering or burning may sometimes occur.

- Skin color may change. This may last for several months or may be permanent.

- Patients can return to work and regular activities the same day.

- Direct exposure to the sun should be avoided for two weeks, and sunscreen should be used for at least six weeks (exposure to the sun or tanning beds can increase the possibility of hyperpigmentation).

More than one treatment is usually necessary to achieve the desired result.

Afterword

Sage Advice

It is easy to feel overwhelmed with all of the choices and all of the planning. We suggest that you take this information in small bites, so that it is easier to digest. We'd like to leave you with some of the highlights to making a safe and informed choice so that you are well prepared and comfortable with whatever decision you make. Cosmetic surgery isn't for everyone—it's not a quick fix, nor a guarantee of success or happiness. When the decision to have cosmetic surgery is entered into sensibly, it can be a wonderfully rewarding experience. Many patients report that it is the lack of information that contributed most to their unfavorable experiences. Our objective is to give you a solid, broad base of information about an often misunderstood subject. You can build on this base as you research your options. In the interest of summarizing a lot of information, the following points bear repeating.

Checking Credentials

If you do your own legwork, rather than using an information and referral company, make sure you call to check on items such as state licensing, board certification, or surgical facility accreditation. It would be worthless to gather your information and not follow through, especially since there are resources available.

Patient Compliance

Consider postponing or avoiding cosmetic surgery altogether if you feel that you cannot comply with your physician's instructions. If you cannot commit to the "downtime" required for cosmetic surgery, no matter how minimal, you are not a good cosmetic surgery candidate. The pace of our lives continues to move at warp speed. Tools like computers, car phones, and e-mail make us forget that there are some things in life that take plain, old-fashioned time. Resarching, undergoing, and recovering from cosmetic surgery is one of them.

Support from Others

For many different reasons, your spouse or significant other may not be supportive of your decision. If the lack of support will interfere with your recovery (i.e., cooking dinner, cleaning house, childcare, stress), you may want to postpone your decision. As an option, when dealing with household matters, you may wish to contract for household assistance during your recovery. For any emotional aspects, seek professional advice.

Your Doctor

Be sure to choose a physician with whom you feel comfortable and whom you trust. Do not base your decision solely on how much he charges or because someone you know went to him. That physician may not be the best choice for your needs. When you have selected your physician it is of utmost importance that you disclose your complete medical history, including any previous cosmetic procedures (for example, chemical peels), and any personal habits (such as drinking, smoking, or drugs—prescribed or illicit). All of these factors greatly affect your health, safety, and healing. Find out if the facility where your procedure is being performed is accredited and has state-of-the-art life support systems.

Recovery

During your recovery period do whatever is necessary to alleviate any stress and don't be afraid to ask for help. While recovering, you are not sick, but you do need to take it easy. If you have children, be reminded of the demands for their care, and plan for help during the initial healing period. You may want to consider a private-duty nurse to assist you, especially in the first twenty-four to forty-eight hours after surgery. Even if you have a caregiver (spouse, friend, etc.), no one can stay awake for the entire forty-eight-hour period in which most physicians require ice compresses to be applied (usually twenty minutes every hour). And you need your rest! Your physician's office should be able to direct you to someone, or there are numerous home care or companion care companies that can meet those needs. Healing times provided throughout this book are averages. Recovery for you could possibly be slower than the norms. There may be a need for additional assistance, and/or the initial healing period may be extended. Be flexible.

If your household situation is such that you feel you would not be able to take it easy, consider staying in a hotel (with your caregiver) or at a friend's— someone who is willing to assist with your medical and recovery needs.

Complications

At any sign of a complication, call your physician's office immediately. Keloid or hypertrophic scarring requires immediate attention by your physician. If your physician is in another city, ask for a referral close to home so that you can receive regular treatments. Follow the physician's instructions to the letter. If you don't understand them, do not call a friend—call the physician's office and ask for an explanation until you do understand.

The End Result

Now is the time for realized expectations and jubilant celebrations. Every day we get to see the wonders of cosmetic surgery, and we never tire of it. It is absolutely awe-inspiring as to what can be accomplished with modern medicine in the field of plastic/cosmetic surgery. You were beautiful when you went in (because beauty is not just skin deep) and now you're even better. If you are like us at Cosmetic Surgery Consultants, who are also cosmetic surgery patients, we're glad we made the decision, and we will do it again! Best wishes while *exploring the possibilities!*

Appendix

Let Us Know What You Think

Thank you for letting us be a part of your cosmetic surgery decision. Our objective is to have you "look before you leap" because leaping wisely can bring you great satisfaction. This can become one of the most exciting and rewarding decisions you'll ever make.

As the field of cosmetic surgery advances at lightning speed, we want to be on the forefront, delivering timely, topical, and accurate information. To assist with this task, we invite you to share your experiences, thoughts, or comments. You can do so in any manner you wish—either by telephone, fax, or e-mail. Thank you again for your confidence.

Cosmetic Surgery Consultants
Your Cosmetic Surgery Consumer Advocate
4343 Shallowford Road, Suite B-5
Marietta, GA 30062

Telephone: 770-552-3223
Fax: 770-552-9054
e-mail: explore@cscfirst.com
Web site: www.safecosmeticsurgery.com

Please visit our Web site often. We will be continuously adding exciting features such as cosmetic surgery procedure information, a national physician locator of screened and credentialed surgeons, a call-in consultation center where you can talk with a trained consultant, a shopping center for qualified products at preferred pricing, chats, forums, message boards, and much more. We plan to be the leading resource for all your cosmetic/plastic surgery and aesthetic interests.

About the Author

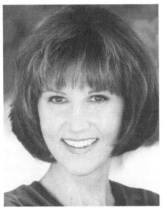

Patricia Burgess, founder and CEO of Cosmetic Surgery Consultants (CSC), has over seventeen years of healthcare marketing, quality management, and business development experience. She began her healthcare career in 1982 as an account representative in the managed care industry with the nation's leading HMO, Aetna/U.S. Healthcare. In 1986, she formed Group Benefit Services, a healthcare brokerage and employee benefit consulting practice. Seeing a trend toward alternative care in 1987, she founded Managed Healthcare Options, a chiropractic HMO, which was acquired by a national chiropractic healthcare company in 1997. Pat has a reputation for leading-edge healthcare projects in which public awareness, consumer advocacy, and added value are her objectives.

Pat's healthcare experience has contributed greatly to the structure of CSC, a specialized information and referral company for individuals considering cosmetic surgery. As a cosmetic surgery patient herself, Pat recognized the need for a resource to assist men and women in making safe and informed decisions. CSC is currently the only company in the United States to apply formal screening and credentialing standards to cosmetic surgeons. Her company's mission is to create the benchmark for quality in an unregulated industry where just about anyone with a medical degree can perform cosmetic surgery.

See Pat's before and after pictures on the next page.

Pat Burgess, Before and After

BEFORE

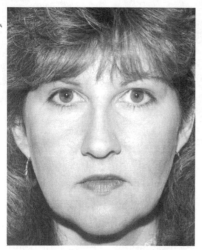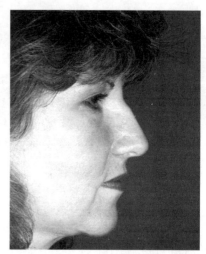

AFTER

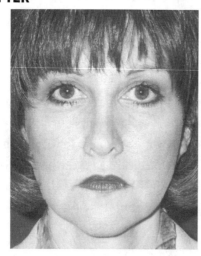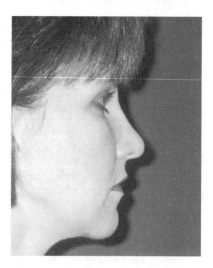

In 1994, at age 37, Pat had a face-lift, brow lift, rhinoplasty (nose reshaping), lower blepharoplasty (lower eyelid surgery), and otoplasty. The "after" pictures were taken five years after the initial surgery. All of the procedures were performed at the same time. Additional planned procedures are liposuction, skin resurfacing, and another face-lift.

Resources

The information provided by these organizations varies from state to state.

STATE LICENSING BOARDS

	Telephone	Fax
Alabama State Board of Medical Examiners	334-242-4116	334-242-4155
Alaska State Medical Board	907-269-8160	907-269-8156
Arizona State Board of Medical Examiners	602-255-3751	602-255-1848
Arkansas State Medical Board	501-296-1802	501-296-1805
California State Medical Board	916-263-2389	916-263-2387
Colorado State Medical Examining Board	303-894-7690	303-894-7692
Connecticut Medical Examining Board	860-509-7579	860-509-8457
Delaware Board of Medical Practice	302-739-4522	302-739-2711
District of Columbia Board of Medicine	202-727-5365	202-727-4087
Florida Board of Medicine	904-488-0595	904-487-9622
Georgia Composite State Board of Medical Examiners	404-656-3913	404-656-9723
Guam Board of Medical Examiners (dial 011 first)	671-475-0251	671-477-4733
Hawaii Board of Medical Examiners	808-586-2708	808-586-2689
Idaho State Board of Medicine	208-334-2822	208-334-2801
Illinois Department of Professional Regulation	312-814-4500	312-814-1837
Indiana Health Professions Service Bureau	317-232-2960	317-233-4236
Iowa State Board of Medical Examiners	515-281-5171	515-242-5908
Kansas State Board of Healing Arts	913-296-7413	913-296-0852
Kentucky Board of Medical Licensure	502-429-8046	502-429-9923
Louisiana State Board of Medical Examiners	504-524-6763	504-568-8893
Maine Board of Registration in Medicine	207-287-3605	207-287-6590
Maryland Board of Physician Quality Assurance	410-764-4777	410-764-2478
	Toll Free 800-492-6836	
Massachusetts Board of Registration in Medicine	617-727-3086	617-451-9568
Michigan Board of Medicine	517-335-0918	517-373-2179
Minnesota Board of Medical Practice	612-617-2130	612-617-2166
Mississippi State Board of Medical Licensure	601-987-3079	601-987-4159
Missouri State Board of Registration for the Healing Arts	573-751-0098	573-751-3166
Montana Board of Medical Examiners	406-444-4284	406-444-1667
Nebraska State Board of Examiners in Medicine & Surgery	402-471-2115	402-471-3577
Nevada State Board of Medical Examiners	775-688-2559	775-688-2321
New Hampshire Licensing Board of Medicine	603-271-1203	603-271-6702
New Jersey State Board of Medical Examiners	609-826-7100	609-984-3930
New Mexico State Board of Medical Examiners	505-827-7317	505-827-7377

	Telephone	Fax
New York Board of Professional Medical Conduct	518-474-8357	518-474-4471
New York State Board of Medicine	518-474-3841	518-486-4846
North Carolina Board of Medicine	919-326-1100	919-326-1131
North Dakota State Board of Medical Examiners	701-328-6500	701-328-6505
Ohio State Medical Board	614-466-3934	614-728-8946
Oklahoma State Board of Medicine Licensure & Supervision	405-848-2189	405-848-8240
Oregon Board of Medical Examiners	503-229-5770	503-229-6543
Pennsylvania State Board of Medicine	717-783-2381	717-783-7769
Puerto Rico Board of Medical Examiners	787-782-8989	787-782-8733
Rhode Island Board of Licensure and Discipline	401-222-3855	401-222-2158
South Carolina, State Board of Medical Examiners of	803-896-4500	803-896-4515
Tennessee State Board of Medical Examiners	615-532-4384	615-532-5369
Texas State Board of Medical Examiners	512-305-7130	512-305-7008
Utah Physicians Licensing Board	801-530-6628	801-530-6511
Vermont Board of Medical Practice	802-828-2673	802-828-5450
Virginia Board of Medicine	804-662-9908	804-662-9943
Virgin Islands Board of Medical Examiners	340-776-8311	340-777-4001
Washington Department of Health	360-664-8480	360-586-4573
West Virginia State Board of Medicine	304-558-2921	304-558-2084
Wisconsin Medical Examiners Board	608-266-2811	608-261-7083
Wyoming Board of Medicine	307-778-7053	307-778-2069

FACILITY ACCREDITATION ORGANIZATIONS

American Association for Accreditation of Ambulatory
Plastic Surgery Facilities (AAAAHC)... 847-949-6058
American Association for Ambulatory Healthcare (AAAHC) 847-676-9610
Federated Ambulatory Surgery Association 703-836-8808
Joint Commission on Accreditation of Healthcare Organizations (JCAHO) 630-792-5000
State—Medicare.. Contact your State Medicare office

PROFESSIONAL SOCIETIES AND ORGANIZATIONS

American Academy of Cosmetic Surgery
Web site: www.cosmeticsurgery.org....................................... 312-527-6713
American Academy of Facial Plastic and Reconstructive Surgeons
Web site: www.facial-plastic-surgery.org.................................. 202-842-4500
American Board of Anesthesiology.. 203-522-9857
American Board of Dermatology
Web site: www.abderm.org.. 313-874-1088
American Board of Medical Specialties (ABMS)
Web site: www.abms.org 800-776-2378
American Board of Facial Plastic and Reconstructive Surgery
Web site: www.abfprs.org.. 703-549-3223

American Board of Plastic Surgery/American Society of Aesthetic Plastic Surgeons
Web site: www.surgery.org 215-587-9322
American Society for Dermatologic Surgery 708-330-0230
American Society of Plastic and Reconstructive Surgeons (ASPRS)
Web site: www.plasticsurgery.org 847-228-9900
California Medical Association
Web site: www.cmanet.org 415-882-5131

CONSUMER RESOURCES

American College of Surgeons
Web site: www.facs.org 312-202-5000
American Medical Association
Web site: www.ama-assn.org 312-464-5000
Physician Data Licensing 312-464-6201
Anesthesia Patient Safety Foundation 412-281-9484
Federation of State Medical Boards
Web site: www.fsmb.org
Institute for Safe Medical Practices
Web site: www.ismp.org
The Public Citizen (Ralph Nader's consumer action group formed in 1971)
Web site: www.citizen.org
Quackwatch
Web site: www.quackwatch.com

PATIENT FINANCING COMPANIES

Cooperative Images 877-THATLOOK
Elite Physician Services 423-296-8122
Jayhawk Medical Acceptance 972-392-5600
MedCash Health Systems 800-800-5820
PulseCard 913-345-2547
Unicorn Financial Services 602-396-9966

References

We have attempted to reference sources that were published most recently. Older works are not necessarily out of date and may provide a perspective about cosmetic surgery for that time period. However, since the field of cosmetic surgery changes so rapidly, we chose to utilize the most recent sources we could locate.

Accreditation Handbook for Ambulatory Health Care. Skokie, Ill.: Accreditation Association for Ambulatory Health Care, 1998.

Alster, Tina, M.D., and Lydia Preston. *Cosmetic Laser Surgery.* Brooklyn, N.Y.: Alliance Publishing, 1997.

Barry, Dianna. *Nips and Tucks.* Santa Monica, Calif.: General Publishing Group, 1996.

Bransford, Helen. *Welcome to Your Facelift.* New York: Doubleday, 1997.

Davis, Kathy. *Reshaping the Female Body.* New York: Routledge, 1995.

Henry, Kimberly A., M.D., and Penny S. Hickman. *The Plastic Surgery Sourcebook.* Los Angeles: Lowell House, 1997.

McCabe, John. *Plastic Surgery Hopscotch.* Santa Monica, Calif.: Carmania Books, 1995.

McCollough, E. Gaylon, M.D. *Plastic Surgery* (Patient Handbook). 4th ed. Birmingham, Ala.: McCollough Plastic Surgery Clinic, 1993.

Nash, Joyce. *What Your Doctor Can't Tell You about Cosmetic Surgery.* Oakland, Calif.: New Harbinger Publications, Inc., 1995.

Perry, Arthur, M.D., and Robin Levinson. *Are You Considering Cosmetic Surgery?* New York: Avon Health, 1997.

Wolf, Naomi. *The Beauty Myth.* New York: William Morrow, 1991.

Yoho, Robert A., M.D., and Judy Brandy-Yoho. *A New Body in One Day.* Studio City, Calif.: First House Press, 1997.

Patrick Hudson, M.D.'s Web site: www.phudson.com

California Medical Association's (CMA Net) Web site: www.cmanet.org

American Board of Medical Specialties' (ABMS) Web site: www.abms.org

American Board of Plastic Surgery/American Society of Aesthetic Plastic Surgeons' Web site: www.surgery.org

American Society of Plastic and Reconstructive Surgeons' (ASPRS) Web site: www.plasticsurgery.org

American Academy of Facial Plastic and Reconstructive Surgeons' Web site: www.facial-plastic-surgery.org

Index